HIDDEN AFFECTS
IN
SOMATIC DISORDERS

HIDDEN AFFECTS
IN SOMATIC DISORDERS:
PSYCHOANALYTIC PERSPECTIVES
ON ASTHMA, PSORIASIS,
DIABETES, CEREBROVASCULAR
DISEASE, AND OTHER DISORDERS

LUIS A. CHIOZZA

Psychosocial Press
Madison, Connecticut

Library of Congress Cataloging-in-Publication Data

Chiozza, Luis A.
    Hidden affects in somatic disorders : psychoanalytic perspectives
  on asthma, psoriasis, diabetes, cerebrovascular disease, and other
  disorders / Luis A. Chiozza.
        p.   cm.
    Includes bibliographical references.
    ISBN 1-887841-16-4
    1. Medicine, Psychosomatic. 2. Psychoanalysis. I. Title.
    [DNLM: 1. Psychophysiologic Disorders--etiology.
  2. Psychophysiologic Disorders--complications. 3. Disease-
  -etiology. 4. Psychoanalytic Theory.   WM 90 C539h 1998]
  RC49.C437 1998
  616.08--dc21
  DNLM/DLC
  for Library of Congress   98-15126
                                                                 CIP

Manufactured in the United States of America

CONTENTS

INTRODUCTION

L. A. Chiozza

The core of this book is formed by six papers written in the Research Department of the Weizsaecker Center for Medical Consultations in Buenos Aires, Argentina. The authors, a group of psychoanalysts seeking to create a center for medical consultation where diagnostic and therapeutic assistance for the patient is based on clinical criteria including the psychoanalytic viewpoint, founded the Weizsaecker Center nearly twenty years ago. At that time, most of our research, teaching, and scientific meetings were conducted at the Center for Research in Psychoanalysis and Psychosomatic Medicine (CIMP), founded four years earlier. There, psychoanalysts of different generations shared (even if sometimes only temporarily) the theoretical framework that forms our view of psychoanalysis and medicine.

Seven years ago, we opened the Foundation for the Psychosomatic Study of the Organic Patient (FEPSEO). Three years ago, we centralized our outpatient-centered efforts—research, treatment, and teaching—in the Weizsaecker Center. Here, we established the Research Department, where the papers in this book were written, and the Sigmund Freud Institute of Metahistorical Psychoanalysis, which is dedicated to the teaching of psychoanalysis.

The term "metahistorical" defines our orientation in psychoanalysis, which is based on a particular conception of history that permeates Freud's thought, however implicitly. In the first chapter, "The construction of a psychoanalytic history," we deal immediately with metahistorical theory because it helps us to show that histories can be constructed in different ways, each of which implies a distinctive type of thought.

The Research Department began by organizing eight groups of psychoanalysts, most of them also physicians, whose objective was to discover different *specific fantasies*. Later, new groups and subjects of investigation joined them. The central chapters of this book are the first papers this project produced whose level of elaboration merited publication. These papers were extensively reviewed in a seminar organized for that purpose in 1990. The idea that there are unconscious fantasies specific to different organic dysfunctions or disorders can be seen throughout our work from its beginning in 1963, when we published *Psychoanalysis of Hepatic Disorders* (Chiozza, 1963).

In the last chapter of this book, we review the history of these ideas on the basis of a minutely detailed study of Freud's works, but it is best to preview an essential aspect of that history at this point. In Freud's psychoanalytic writings, we find two different epistemologies: one, derived from the natural science of his time, is explicit; the other is implicit and represents the way of thinking that led to psychoanalysis. It has been consolidated over the last fifty years by "new" thought in the traditional disciplines (physics or linguistics, for example); it also pertains directly to new disciplines such as genetic engineering and cybernetics. In the first epistemology, body and soul as well as time and space are different ontological realities existing beyond consciousness. Nature is sharply differentiated from culture, and the psychical world is formed, *from* matter and *in* living matter, when such matter acquires sufficient organization to include a nervous system or some type of "brain."

In this epistemology, the universe is structured "geometrically" like logic, while reason, which is structured as a secondary process in our preconscious, is the zenith of intelligence. In this theoretical framework, knowing is nearly the same as knowing the cause and being able to explain the mechanism that causes an effect.

The other epistemology holds that body and soul as well as space and time are *notions*, categories established by consciousness to describe a reality that is in itself incomprehensible. In this epistemology, in which "body" is what is perceived by the senses and "psyche" is what possesses meaning, the myth acquires proximity to the object of knowledge, which is no less than what science pursues. The basic question is not whether the strike of a thunderbolt is "really" a punishment. The epistemological change consists in no longer thinking that lightning is "really" an electromagnetic force. Both myth and science are different maps of an inaccessible territory. Logic is no longer a quality of the universe but a temporary state in the progressive evolution of the human intellect; among the instruments with which we apprehend reality, poetry and mathematics hold similar epistemological value. The relation between symbol and referent becomes as significant as the relation between cause and effect. Therefore, the nature and objective of our investigation lead us to study both the physical disorders of the body and the historical vicissitudes of psychical life. We believe that our observations throughout years of work at the Weizsaecker Center confirm what we foresaw theoretically as early as 1963: each particular physical alteration that we can define as characteristic and universal, be it physiological or pathological, gives shape to an unconscious meaning—"its" own particular meaning—that is as characteristic and universal as the disorder per se.

Freud held that affects are equivalents of hysterical attacks and that they are characteristic, universal, and congenital. In 1976, when we wrote *Body, Affect and Language* (Chiozza, 1976), we went further by adding a new concept to the idea of a specific unconscious fantasy inherent in each of the different bodily forms, functions, and physical disorders.

At that time, we thought that displacement "within" the "innervation code" of an affect leads the process of discharge to deform the configuration of that affect so that when it enters consciousness deprived of its emotional meaning, it becomes a somatic process. Therefore, we can say that bodily disorders *conceal* affects, in the sense that disorders are discharge processes that substitute and avoid a certain development of affect. When we attempt to discover the specific unconscious fantasies involved in a certain physical function or disorder, we use not only the "clinical" material that we can extract from a psychoanalytic session or from a pathobiography, but also everyday linguistic expressions, the etymological origins of the words used, myths, literature, and all forms of symbolic activity available to us. We seek a meaning that is embedded in more than one of the above-specified sources and can therefore be identified as the characteristic fantasy involved in a certain bodily function, or as the specific "script" of a given physical alteration.

We wish to acknowledge a debt of gratitude to all those colleagues in our Center who, though not listed as authors of this book, contributed their cooperation, companionship, and constant stimulation to its materialization.

The road we are traveling together, sharing moments of enthusiasm and of despair, passes through a territory that upsets our unconscious epistemological "beliefs" and is therefore viewed with curiosity and misunderstanding by those who approach our work without going into it deeply. Living as we do in a world in constant acceleration added to the detrimental prejudice in favor of "easy" reading, caution leads us to accept that not all our readers will decide to put in time in studying and reflecting on what they are reading. In view of that caution, we have spared no effort in our attempt to write clearly, although we have not forgotten what Weizsaecker (1950a) stated: ". . . when something inherently difficult is rendered in an easy form . . . ," a falsification is committed. "The most important things are certainly simple, yet difficult."

1

THE CONSTRUCTION
OF A PSYCHOANALYTIC HISTORY

L. A. Chiozza

I. The Clinical History

The doctor asks questions in order to find out what happened, which means that the doctor requests a history. The doctor also uses methods derived from physics to examine the patient, in order to gather data on a state called current; from these, he infers the characteristics of a former state and the possibilities for a future state. By including the temporal dimension in the work of exploring matter, the doctor is using a conception of "linear" time that derives from the exercise of logical thought, and therefore, the clinical history is in a broad sense basically chronological. It is a series of facts that enable the conception and interpretation of the evolution of a process in which an antecedent cause and a consequent effect are postulated.

During the treatment of Anna O., Breuer discovered that his patient's hysterical attacks were relieved when she was able to remember certain traumatic events. A decade later, Freud, as a practicing neurologist on his way to developing psychoanalysis, remarked that his clinical histories were beginning to read more like literary works than neurological contributions.

We find another type of history whose essential meaning does not necessarily emerge from what happened first and what happened afterwards. It is a history that reaches the conscious not as history but as a current drama, because it is still alive in each action and is ongoing in an eternal present. This history can be narrated anytime and anywhere, since it is forever being repeated, as if it were new, as in the "once upon a time . . ." of fairy tales in which everything happens in "a" time that is "the first" only because the conscious forgets what memory "knows": that "this" time is simultaneously "again."

Thus, the image of circular time is created, not so much because of the idea of eternal recurrence but because of the fact that in this type of history, as in fights between siblings or the dispute between Laius and Oedipus, it is impossible to know "who started it": the effect can be interpreted as the cause of its own cause.

From these considerations, it follows that two different clinical histories can be written about the event that led the patient to see the doctor. One history will interpret it as a current state originating in past causes and will describe the background whose concatenation has led to the present, since this one is based on the idea that it is the position of the event in a chronology that grants or denies the possibility of an influence. The other history, interpreting the event as a sign in a cryptic language that is expressing a drama the patient is hiding from himself or herself, will put together a plot that includes that apparently accidental episode as a coherent part of a meaning that permeates the whole biography. Although the two histories employ different conceptions of time, each is equally legitimate; it has been a long time since we stopped considering mythical thought to be primitive and inadequate and therefore inferior to logic.

II. THE ACTUALITY[1] OF THE PRESENT AND THE HISTORY OF THE PAST

We have learned that "actuality" and "history" are two ways of representing the same reality to ourselves, acting in the physical universe as an interrelation of forces that operate in "geometric" space and appearing on the stage of history as a drama that occurs in a "linguistic" time, free of the inevitability of sequence. Once we have grasped that a history never consists in the facts that have really happened but, precisely, in their meaning,[2] we also comprehend that access to a "past" meaning depends entirely on the continuity of that meaning in the present. A history can only narrate what is alive in the present, in the sense that it has not finished occurring. Psychoanalytic experience confirms that just as Freud said, we repeat in our behavior precisely what is painful for us to remember; therefore, when we construct a history, we attribute a time, a place, and a sequence to the scene that condenses the meaning of current acts.

In thinking that history resides not in the mere description of a series of acts but in the meaning that links them, we give a new meaning to

---

[1]In Spanish *actualidad* implies both an "actual," "real," action and "present time."

[2]The first type of history, it must be noted, is also constructed by using the meanings of what has happened (interpretations) and not on the basis of "what really happened."

our concepts of historical "truth." Even if we admit that "what really happened" exists as an ultimate referent, we also know that, just as Pirandello shows in his "Six Characters in Search of an Author," it is an unapproachable event. When Freud, in the case history of the "Wolf-Man" (1918b) and in his *Introductory Lectures on Psychoanalysis* (1916–1917) questioned the reality value of the reconstruction of the primary scenes witnessed in childhood, he concluded that the impossibility of separating the true from the false in no way diminishes the value of these scenes in coming to understand current psychical reality, a reality in which some fragment of that unknown event that happened at some time always remains.

The "true" history is therefore the one that is constructed, applying a rigorous method, through the very process of its interpretation, through the inevitable confluence of what is interpreted and the interpreter's view, since a part of the "past" unknown reality remains alive in the current present of both.

III. INQUIRE, INVESTIGATE, AND ASCERTAIN

We tend to use the word "History" with a capital "H" to refer to the science called "history" that is still generally subject to the rational idea of time ordered as a sequence of successive events. The word "history"[3] with a small "h" refers, on the other hand, to the narration, story, or account whose construction admits other conceptions of time. While History proposes an objective investigation, history is made with imagination and memory. However, psychoanalysis and also new theories in physics have undermined the basis for this distinction by holding that the possibility of remembering is the very basis of the notion of time, thereby eliminating the possibility of History per se. Thus, history acquires citizenship in the territory of science.

Psychoanalysis also demonstrates that the differences between testimony, based on memory, and imagination, arising from fantasy, blur in the unconscious.

The psychoanalytic procedure that enables us to construct a history involves three functions, namely, inquiring (in Spanish, *averiguar*, whose root is *verdad*, truth), investigating, and ascertaining (in Spanish, *acertar*, which means "to hit the target" and shares the same root as "certain" and "truthful"). If we restore its original meaning to the word *averiguar*, i.e., "search for truth," and if we consider truth to be "that which reason cannot refute," then we can hold that to inquire about a history in the rigorous or strict sense is to distinguish in it, by means of reason, what we consider to be true.

---

[3]In Spanish we use the word "history" to refer both to one's life story and to history as a science. In light of the explanation that follows, we continue to use the word "history" throughout.

The word "investigate" originally meant to pursue the traces, the lasting impression, of a past event. Recovering the original meaning of the term, to investigate a history is to reconstruct it on the basis of what is preserved in the current present. It is important to note that the investigation progresses because of the interpretation and, more importantly, because it takes the vanguard and makes perception of the traces possible. It is also important to underscore that the kind of interpretation we have in mind is one in which imagination is combined with the rigor of a method that involves and at the same time transcends reason.

The word *acertar* means "to hit the target," and we use it now because we need to differentiate between what is true and what hits the target. To find a history is therefore suddenly to find ourselves face to face with it: that special moment when our mind replaces a series of "and so?" with the exclamation "aha!" Hence, the "global" perception-interpretation of a universal and eternal leitmotiv. It is a theme that exists within us whole and preformed, often repressed and unconscious. Its existence opens our only access to that mysterious process that we call "realizing the importance of a meaning."

If we wish to express, on the terrain of physical symbolization, the process by which a history is constructed, we can say that it is necessary to inquire with a clear head, "to have the stamina"[4] to investigate and the "heart" (courage) to open the way to the hunch or presentiment of having hit the target. Furthermore, these three "functions" converge when evaluating the degree of credibility we can assign to a history.

IV. INTRIGUE

We must discuss yet another question. The construction of a history requires a reason, and the reason for every history is ultimately intrigue. The word "intrigue" originally meant an entanglement, and we may suppose that it refers to a kind of tangle in which the vacillating potential for contrary and very important meanings persists. The intrigue is undone when the history culminates and the meaning is elucidated.

Since universal themes seem to be numerous, the possibilities for generating different intrigues also seem to be infinite. However, the psychoanalytic study of "primary scenes" and "primary fantasies" has been able to refer the enormous kinds of possible vicissitudes to a few basic nuclei, at the same time confirming the idea that the Oedipus legend is the nuclear complex. If we take this perspective to study what the diverse intrigues have in common, we discover that they all have two phases, moments, or situations that we can name in a thousand different

---

[4]In Spanish, *hígado*, "liver."

ways, making them infinitely complex. Every history involves success and failure, guilt and expiation, or, to say it in the original oedipal terms, incest and castration. In the same way, each intrigue involves joy and pain, and when the iterative circle is broken off and time stretches out in a linear course, the story will be sad or not according to which of the terms is temporarily placed at the end.

2

AN APPROACH TO THE SPECIFIC UNCONSCIOUS FANTASIES IN COMMON PSORIASIS

L. A. Chiozza, S. Grinspon, E. Lanfri

I. Psoriasis: Basic Concepts

A. Normal Skin

Physiology considers the skin a "border organ," demarcating the internal and external environments and regulating exchange between them. In addition to forming a protective shield without which life would be impossible, it is a sense organ, inasmuch as its nerve endings are mediators for four types of sensations: touch, pain, cold, and heat. Its embryological origin is mixed (ecto- and mesodermal), and it comprises three tissue layers: epidermis, dermis, and hypodermis.

The epidermis is a multistratified epithelium consisting basically of two layers: the germinative Malpighian layer and the corneal layer, the end product of the keratinization process. The corneal layer is formed of amorphous elements that desquamate continually. The deepest cell layers form the "barrier zone" regulating the transfer of chemical substances and infectious agents toward the dermis and preventing rapid loss of water from the epidermis into the environment. In the mucous and semi-mucous membranes, there is no corneal layer. One of the most important functions of the epidermis is to produce keratin, a protein found in the dead cells of the corneal layer. The epidermis is a kinetic system in which cells divide, migrate, differentiate, and die. It has been estimated that turnover of the epidermis takes approximately 30 days in humans. The process of desquamation and renewal is imperceptible and continuous.

7

The dermis is a fibrous tissue, much thicker than the epidermis; it contains two types of specialized structures: the corneal (hair and nails) and the glandular (sebaceous and sudoriferous). The functions of the dermis are protection and also provision of the ducts and support necessary for the cutaneous vascular system.

The hypodermis, or subcutaneous fat layer, exercises various functions: thermal insulation, trauma absorption, and storage of energy in the form of fat.

B. General Characteristics of Psoriasis

Robert Williams, an English doctor, first described the illness in 1808. Dermatologists (Magnin, 1977) describe different varieties of psoriasis: common, inverted, pustulous, arthropathic, and erythrodermal. We discuss the common form, since it is the most typical. Common psoriasis is a chronic skin disease that develops in capricious and unpredictable ways in separate outbreaks after varying periods of latency and includes intervals of complete remission.

Common psoriasis affects men just as frequently as women, but Caucasians more than individuals of other races. Onset occurs at any age, and the average age at onset is 27. The condition was thought to be rare in newborns or during early childhood, but recent investigations indicate that 2% of psoriasis patients had the disease during the first two years of life.

C. Etiology

Current investigations (Panconesi et al., 1984) stress that human skin is a far more complex organ than previously acknowledged. According to these studies, some metabolic functions of epidermal cells are closely related to the defenses of the immune system. From this viewpoint, psoriasis is currently considered an immuno-allergic disease.

The etiology of psoriasis is unknown. Some studies (Fitzpatrick et al., 1979; Panconesi et al., 1984) support the hypothesis of multifactorial inheritance involving polygenic and environmental factors. They underscore the importance in psoriasis of the main human leukocyte antigens (HLA located on chromosome 6). Panconesi and co-workers (1984) observed functional defects in, and reduced numbers of, T lymphocytes and increase in circulating IgA and IgE and HLA-dependent immune complexes.

D. Clinical Description and Localization

Psoriasis is an erythematous-squamous disease characterized by hyperplasia and greatly accelerated renewal of the epidermis. It is evidenced in the form of well-defined and sometimes slightly raised pink or red patches, covered by scales in varying quantities. There is generally no itching. Lesions, which nearly always are symmetrical in distribution, are usually found on the scalp (parietal-mastoid and occipital areas, without hair loss), elbows, knees, sacrum and coccyx, palms and soles, fingernails, or toenails. Oral lesions are rare. Lesions can affect the trunk, the legs, and any part of the skin surface except for the face and areas of the skin in which sebaceous glands are found. On the joints, the disease mainly affects sites where the skin is stretched (Magnin, 1977).

The first outbreak of the disease is associated with, and takes place in proximity to, a superficial cutaneous trauma: a burn, a cut, a scrape, contact-induced allergic dermatitis, drug-produced allergic exanthema, chicken pox, measles, and the like.

E. DIFFERENTIAL DIAGNOSIS

Scraping the patches with a scalpel yields valuable diagnostic data since the manner in which the scales and other layers detach varies according to the type of erythematous-squamous disorder. The pattern of detachment seen in psoriasis is as follows: (a) dry and powdery scales (sign of the stearin candle) detach; (b) a film formed by the condensation of the last corneal layers lifts off; (c) under these a red and shiny surface with tiny congested dots (bloody dew) can be seen; and (d) if scraping is continued, exoserosis and purpura come into view (Gatti & Cardama, 1963).

F. PATHOGENESIS

The following sequence is observed:

1. Thickening of the epidermis (acanthosis).
2. Elongation of dermal papillae.
3. Increased mitotic activity (more discernible in the epidermis): the median psoriatic germinative cell reproduces every 37.5 hours, instead of every 152 hours as in normal epidermis. Further, normal epidermal cell mitosis takes place only in the single layer of basal cells, while in psoriasis it is found in three layers of cells.
4. Parakeratose hyperkeratosis: thickening of the corneal layer is due to the increased number of proliferating germinative cells. It has been demonstrated that the cells of the corneal layer have retained their nuclei (parakeratosis), because the rapidly accelerated exit of cells from the germinal zone has impeded complete keratination.

5. Absence or decrease in thickness of the granular layer: the thickness of the granular layer is often inversely proportionate to the rate of epidermal proliferation.
6. An inflammatory infiltrate into the subcapillary dermis is always observed.
7. Proliferation of subepidermal blood vessels and increased blood circulation is then seen (Magnin, 1977; Fitzpatrick et al., 1979).

The fact that the pathologic changes of psoriasis are expressed in both the dermis and the epidermis has led to controversy. For some, the disease begins in the dermis and for others in the epidermis. Braun-Falco, quoted by E. Farber and E. Van Scott (1980), suggested that the dermis and epidermis react together as an integrated system in the development of psoriasis.

G. TREATMENT

Currently, no treatment achieves permanent cure of psoriasis. The lesions usually respond to any of several treatments the first time they are administered, only to become resistant later. Sometimes it is difficult to determine the cause of improvement. Therapies of long standing are: (1) ultraviolet light; while beneficial in appropriate doses, overexposure provokes worsening; (2) tars; and (3) anthraline. There are newer treatments that must be administered with great care because of the side effects they may cause; these include the use of corticosteroids and of methotrexate. In some clinically severe forms of psoriasis, the use of etretinate has yielded acceptable results.

II. INTRODUCTION TO THE MEANINGS OF THE SKIN

Some authors implicitly used a psychogenetic conception in their work on psoriasis, e.g., Strandberg (1932), Obermayer (1956) and Weiss & English (1949). Although Rof Carballo (1950) shares this conception, he went a step further when he stated that we can think in terms of expressive symbolism in skin diseases. However, he recommends that such interpretations be made only after all somatic etiologies have been ruled out.

Panconesi and other authors (1984) investigated "psychosomatic" problems in dermatology. In reviewing the history of psychosomatic investigation, they found a prevailing tendency to resolve questions of the origin of the illness from a unilateral perspective, either psychogenetic or somatogenetic. They attempted to go beyond these positions by proposing that both the somatic factor and the psychical factor be sought at the same time in each case, in order to determine the cause of the disease. However, their understanding of cutaneous disorders does not transcend the simplistic cause-and-effect way of thinking implicit in the concept of psychogenesis (Shanon in Panconesi et al., 1984). We, on the other hand, hold that the organ, its function, and its disorders have a specific psychological sense or meaning that can be understood in the same way that one understands a language (Chiozza, 1963).

We find two groups of ideas in Freud regarding the skin. One refers to the skin as a contact surface (Freud, 1905d) and the other, to the skin as a barrier (Freud, 1920g). Although different parts of the skin and mucous membrane are special erogenous zones, any sector of skin can act as an erogenous zone, since any and all organs can function as the source of a qualitatively differentiated impulse. Freud (1905d) postulated an impulse to skin contact (with another person), regarding it as an important component of the sex drive.

The second group of ideas is related to what Freud, in "Beyond the pleasure principle" (1920g), called the barrier against stimuli. He referred to the "undifferentiated vesicle" (1920g, p. 26) as a model of primitive life that protects itself by creating a barrier whose external surface is no longer structured like living matter but has become inorganic and acts as a special wrapping or membrane to keep stimuli away. Freud (1923b) also stated that the ego is, above all, a body ego, derived mainly from sensations originating on the surface of the body. In 1927 he added that in addition to representing the surface ("superficies") of the psychical apparatus, the ego may be thought of as the psychical projection of that surface (Freud, 1923b, p. 26, n1).

As a contact surface, the skin is a constant source of sensation and perception. When babies suckle their mothers' breast—in the stage of the pleasure-ego—they tend to consider that this breast is theirs, just as the thumb they suck is. The "pleasure-ego" slowly gives way to the "reality-ego" when a baby discovers that the act of suckling is not accompanied by the same somatic sensation that is experienced on sucking the thumb since, in the latter case, "sucking" and "being sucked" are experienced simultaneously. We must bear in mind the difference between "touching" and "touching oneself" and the relation between these actions and cutaneous perception and sensation.

Paul Schilder (1958) believes that the skin plays an important role in the conformation of the body scheme, which is intimately related to the constitution of the feeling of identity. Children constantly experience sensations that lead them to touch themselves and to induce others to touch them. These contacts provide experiences with the world and enrich their own body image. The construction of the body image is thus based on relationships between the subject and others.

Portmann (1961) postulated that the variations in the external aspect of those organisms which have lost their transparency during phylogenetic development evidence internal variations and constitute the specific manner in which each life form presents itself. He asserted that this form of "self-presentation" always involves a meaning. In this sense, the skin exercises a symbolic function of self-represer.tation of the subject.

In view of the several considerations put forward by the authors we have discussed, we must for our purposes take into account the functions of the skin as a contact surface, as a limiting barrier, as a contribution to the constitution of the feeling of identity in the body scheme, and as an organ capable of exercising the symbolic function of representing the subject's self. We believe that these functions are related to the specific unconscious fantasies associated with the skin organ.

A. THE SKIN AS A CONTACT SURFACE. EROTOGENIC ZONE

Freud (1905d) defined the erogenous zones as those parts of the epidermis or of the mucous membrane which, when acted upon by certain stimuli, produce pleasurable sensations. Both the source and the external stimulus are important for the sensation of pleasure. Referring to the former, Freud (1905d) observed that the state of need is expressed in two different ways: a sensation of unpleasurable tension and a centrally conditioned stimulus or itch that is projected to the skin erogenous zone. As for the external source, he considered the quality of the external stimulus highly influential. In that regard, we cannot overemphasize the importance of intimate, skin-to-skin contact, as expressed in the act of caressing.[1] The first experiences of "skin contact" take place during fetal life and continue during labor, when the uterus presses and stimulates the skin of the fetus and the walls of the birth canal exert pressure on its body. Since the child's skin is such an important system of communication, messages received on this level must be satisfactory in order for growth and development as a human being to take place.

Montagu (cited by Panconesi et al., 1984) considered the skin to be the basic communications system that keeps the baby "in contact." The warmth of the mother's body inaugurates the experience on which the feeling of warmth is modeled. In English, many words and expressions referring to deep-felt sentiment originate in experiences of touching; this word refers on the one hand to the verb, the act of stimulating the skin ("to touch"); on the other hand, as an adjective ("touching"), it describes the emotional involvement, the interest, the tender care, and

---

[1]Etymologically the word "caress" means "an act or gesture expressing affection." It derives from the Latin *carus* (dear). In turn, *carus* derives from *careo* (to lack). The feelings of nostalgia and wishfulness are included in the original idea of *carus*, and this word is thought to come from a form that means "to feel nostalgia." We also know that "nostalgia" is defined as "a desire to return . . ." and derives from the Greek *nostos* (return home) and *algos* (pain). It is widely known that the awakening and development of the child's senses depend partly on the quantity and quality of skin contact the baby has with its mother from the very beginning. This contact provides the baby with varied experiences of pleasure associated with sensations of softness and warmth.

the empathy that a loving mother feels toward her child. We may add that the term "touching" also expresses the double quality of the skin as an organ that both touches and feels.

B. THE SKIN AS A CONTAINER

It is often said that the skin organ acts as a boundary between inside and outside and between body and world. Since it covers the entire body surface and functions physiologically as a wrapper, we may deduce that this function takes on the psychical representation of a container. Basing their thinking on the Freudian ideas we have mentioned, Foks et al. (1969) asserted that the corneal layer can be considered a physical equivalent of the coherent ego, both because of its mediating function between what is external and what is internal to the subject and also because of its function as protection from excitation.

D. Anzieu's (1987) theoretical position is that each psychical function develops from the infrastructure of a physical function. He regards the skin as fundamentally important since, as Freud postulated, it provides the psyche with the representations that constitute the ego and its main functions. D. Anzieu used the term "skin-ego" to denote a psychical configuration formed of the experience of the subject's own skin surface. The child uses that configuration in the early stages of development to represent himself or herself as an ego. When the author described the functions of the skin-ego, he attempted to define the correlations between the organic and the psychical.

D. Anzieu further postulated that the skin-ego is a structure whose universal nature suggests that it is inscribed or "pre-programmed" in the budding psyche; furthermore, he considers the skin a "fact" originally belonging to both the organic and the imaginary orders. These two latter affirmations imply the idea of a body that is originally symbolic; however, D. Anzieu drew his conclusions on the basis of the conception that "the body is that which the psychical functions rest upon" (D. Anzieu, 1987). Our position, in contrast, is that reality in itself is neither physical nor psychical, since "physical" and "psychical" are the attributes our consciousness perceives of as a single unconscious entity, incomprehensible in itself—in a sense analogous to that of a *Ding an sich*, in Kant's terms (Chiozza, 1980). Following this view, we would say that the skin exists as an organ simultaneously with the fantasy of the skin-ego, rather than consider this fantasy a derivative of the already existing organ.

Bick (1968) asserted that the representation of the skin as a container contributes to the integration of the body image, since this representation ensures the cohesion of the parts of the baby's personality initially experienced as lacking integration. This function depends on the introjection of an object experienced as being capable of providing such cohesion. When this happens, appropriate action of the containing object acquires the psychical representation of a "first skin."[2] Bick also stated that disorders of this function can produce the formation of a pseudo-self and acquire, in unconscious fantasy, the representation of a "second skin"; it is evidenced, for example, in behavior that from this viewpoint can be interpreted along the lines of functioning as a "muscular shield." This expression refers to motor hyperactivity acting as a defense against the feeling of lack of integration of the self. Although Bick did not study patients with cutaneous symptoms, his ideas refer to the meanings of the functions and pathologies of the skin.

Rosenfeld (1975), taking up Bick's concepts regarding the containing function the skin acquires in unconscious fantasy, believes that a patient with a skin disorder has two basic unresolved conflicts: one associated with experiences of softness and warmth and the other related to experiences of support and organization of the different parts of the self. We believe, however, that this second conflict is better represented by the alteration of other organic structures, as in, for example, bone disorders (see Chapter VI).

When we consider an individual's skin as a "wrapper," insulating and differentiating the person from his or her surroundings, we assume that the skin is a limit: everything external is the "world" and everything that remains inside is the "ego." However, there is obviously a component of illusion in the feeling of individuality formed on the basis of this assumption, considering that identity is established through identifications that imply a relationship between the subject and his environment, circumstance, or context, a relationship that transcends the framework of the container-contained dichotomy.

The feeling of lack of protection that accompanies situations in which the ego is insufficient as a container leads to defensive reactions that may take the form of hardness and inflexibility in the areas of behavior or character; because of the illusion that we have mentioned, they may be expressed in the skin as, for example, a hyperkeratosis. The patches of hyperkeratosis express the fantasy that they function like the shell of insects, which, as invertebrates, lack an internal skeleton but develop an external structure that provides them with both protection and support (see Chapter VI).

C. The Skin and Identity

The feeling of identity depends on the capacity for recognizing oneself in the peculiarity of one's own form, manner, and style, which implies the capacity for recognizing the difference between what is one's own,

---

[2]We refer here to Bick's idea (1968) that when the experience of the nipple in the baby's mouth and that of the mother holding the baby are combined, this image is experienced as a skin.

what is "familiar," and what is strange (often incorrectly called "foreign," since foreign is the unknown) (Chiozza, 1986c). The recognition of what is one's own also stems from external recognition, which is also closely related to what we show of ourselves to others. Therefore, the other person's gaze contributes to what it means to "feel oneself." Therefore, an individual's body image depends not only on the limits formed by the skin surface, since significant earliest contact with persons in the environment "returns" an image of him- or herself that is essential. The reassurance that comes from those significant beings is experienced as guaranteeing identity, since it establishes the subject's "meaning," assigning value to that person (Chiozza, 1978).

D. Anzieu (1987) indicated that one of the functions of the skin-ego is to ensure the constitution of the "self" in the form of the feeling of existing as a unique being. He established a correlation between this function and the function of protecting individuality exercised by the membrane of an organic cell; it identifies and rejects foreign objects or substances that are similar or complementary to others which it allows to enter. He also noted that remarkably, individual differences in the skin enable us to identify others as objects of attraction or rejection while at the same time providing us with self-affirmation as individuals who recognize the singularity of our own skin. In Spanish there is a saying[3] which refers to a person's positive or negative sensitivity to other people; it is an everyday expression of the function by which we accept what is familiar and reject what is strange. Likewise, in English we say that someone "gets under our skin" when he/she annoys us or becomes an obsession.

We believe it important to stress that the notion that the function of the mental representation of the skin in the body image is to contribute to the feeling of identity is consistent with the results of some biological studies. According to these investigations, the skin has immune functions (Panconesi et al., 1984). The immune system, which protects the organism's own tissues from foreign protein and thereby safeguards its identity, functions by recognizing what belongs, "what is familiar," and differentiating it from what is strange.

---

[3] "*Es una cuestión de piel*," literally translated as "It's a question of skin sensation." In this book, the reader will find frequent references to words which in Spanish have a double meaning. On the one hand, they denote a particular affect, feeling, action, and the like. On the other, they refer to some organ or aspect of the body scheme. Although several languages may make use of such words, the words are, naturally, not used in all languages. In some instances, in order to denote a given referent, we use words of differing etymological meaning which do not refer to the same organs or body functions. At first blush, this may give the impression that the conclusions drawn from the study of the relationship between both meanings in one language are not applicable to another. Therefore, it would appear we cannot establish general conclusions for the relationship between the organs and the body scheme and certain affects, feelings, actions, and the like. However, a closer look allows us to understand that different languages use different partial aspects of a larger and unconscious reality to name it, and therefore all those partial aspects are true representations of the larger reality which is the object of our research.

D. The Skin and its Symbolic Function
   as Self-Representation of the Subject

Portmann (1961) argued that what can be seen is constructed differently from that which remains hidden and is excluded from this "representation"; the image must represent something that is essential in that "more complete other." Any organism, he added, must be viewed while taking into account both its functional as well as its esthetic meaning; the "form" of a living being is a signifying element; therefore, the "representation" of the living form always has a meaning. The opaque covering of higher animals, unlike that of lower animals, which is transparent, is full of designs and colors and other structures of the epidermis that obey the laws of external symmetry. In higher animals, there is a contrast between the internal and the external that is lacking in organisms of a lower order. In higher animals, what is on the outside, like the skin, seems to be there to be seen; it is one of the forms of appearance at the service of self-representation. For this reason, Portmann (1961) stated, "In all cases, variations in appearance attest to variations on the inside." In this sense, we can speak of the skin as an organ of expression.

The self-representative quality of the skin is transferred to human attire, not only when it is used to represent what a subject is but also when it functions to make the subject appear to be something that it is not. An example of this affirmation is the fairytale called "Ass's skin" (Perrault, 1971). In this story, the dresses the princess wears represent what she is; at the same time, when she wears the ass's skin, she does so to appear to be what she is not, a beggar.

A. Garma (1961) believes that clothing and also tatoos originated in the custom in which mothers in certain preliterate societies replaced the fetal membranes covering their newborn infants with clothes and the vernix with tatoos so that the babies would look more as they did when they were inside the womb. Such actions were motivated by a magical fantasy of protection. Secondarily, clothing and tatoos later acquired functions as adornment.

Mimicry is another interesting phenomenon related to the function of self-representation. It is the property that enables some plants and animals to look the same, mainly in color, as other entities, animate or inanimate, in their environment. Some animals change their appearance by changing the characteristics of their skin, with the intention of hiding from predators or, when hunting, from prey (Villée, 1957; Weisz, 1971). The human equivalent to animal mimicry can also be interpreted as a desire to fuse with the other person through projective identification (D. Rosenfeld, 1975). Mankind has lost the capability noted in the phylogenetic record for remarkable and rapid change in appearance. Following Freud's (1923b) statement that the id contains innumerable ego-existences, we believe that this ability remains in the unconscious as archaic behavior that could be reactivated in critical life situations, leading to some skin disorders.

III. THE UNCONSCIOUS FANTASIES EXPRESSED THROUGH PSORIASIS

A. THE FANTASY OF "BEING SKINNED ALIVE"

We can assume that the psoriasis patient has suffered early deprivation of experiences relating to the skin as a contact surface. This "skin-contact" deficiency has left a trace of affective frustration experienced as "hunger for caresses," so that the patient feels an overwhelming need to receive caresses on the skin, or praise as their equivalent, from a valued person.

Korovsky (1978) holds that the psoriasis patient links the onset of the illness to one of a class of traumatic events whose common denominator is the real or fantasied loss of an idealized object. This loss is experienced unconsciously as rejection or desertion, resulting in feelings of humiliation and shame.

We believe that the vasodilation and inflammatory infiltrate of psoriasis, which increase sensitivity and redden the skin, and the desquamation that exposes the surface, express the desertion these patients experience as cruel, as a wound that leaves them "skinned alive" or "flayed." Psoriasis patients fantasy that the idealized object repeatedly attacks, wounds, or causes pain, as, for example, when that object delivers cruel and mocking criticism, sometimes taking the form of sarcasm.[4] These patients cannot bear being criticized by others because they feel it deeply hurts and irritates them. As the linguistic expression describes it, the patients feel they are being "flayed."

B. THE FANTASY OF BEING "SCALED"[5]

The closeness inherent in love relationships makes the psoriasis patient fear that the object might become detached, which makes the patient feel very vulnerable. The feelings of lack of protection and weakness that accompany this fear lead to the fantasy of creating a protective shell as a defense against feeling constantly in danger of getting hurt. We see the hyperkeratosis (thickening of the corneal layer) of psoriasis as the

---

[4]The *Random House Dictionary of the English Language* (1966), New York, N.Y., defines "sarcasm" as "1. harsh or bitter derision or irony. . . ." It derives from the Latin *sarcasmus*, which in turn derives from the Greek *sarkasmos*, from *sarkazein*, which means "to rend (flesh)," "to sneer."

[5]"Scaled" in Spanish also means "to have learned a lesson the hard way" or through punishment.

symbolic expression of the need to have a solid protective barrier, both as a shield against external aggressions and as a container for internal impulses. Psoriasis patients fail to react to what they experience as cruelty from loved ones and feel ashamed of this weakness. Covering themselves with horny patches of psoriasis is an attempt to materialize the desire to become hard and inflexible, wrapped inside a protective shell. This fantasy is also expressed as a personality trait in the form of a superficially "hard" character which is, in fact, "soft."

As for the parakeratosis of psoriasis (accelerated proliferation of immature cells whose ability to form keratin has not matured), it could be interpreted as a representation of the failure of the defense. In this way, it symbolizes that the thick skin[6] of which the shell is made is (as a manifestation of the return of the repressed) an "immature thick skin." The immaturity of these cells would therefore express accelerated and incomplete growth of the ego. The psoriasis patient is enclosed in his own shell and continues to feel helpless and at the same time ashamed of his diseased skin, which in turn leads him/her to feel rejected. The patient also tends to use the fear of rejection to cover up a desire to "keep his/her distance" as a protection from traumatic contact. Since the skin symbolically represents the container function of the ego, the existence of a protective shell in the psoriasis patient helps us to see how this function has been altered.

As noted above, the corneal layer in psoriasis acquires a scaly appearance. We regard the scaly form of psoriasis, in addition to expressing the fantasy of a protective shell, as a symbolic self-representation of the unsuccessful unconscious intention of hiding the patient's shame and humiliation about feeling weak and vulnerable. In this way, the patient tries to "keep up appearances," to present a different image and thus avoid the danger of being found out. This fantasy is implicit in the term "an empty shell": it appears to contain more than it actually does.

The Australian English meaning of the word "scale" is "to cheat; deceive; swindle." This definition, in our opinion, correlates with the unconscious meaning of this disorder and also with these patients' behavior, since they are remarkably suspicious, always alert in situations that they imagine might endanger their most personal traits, which they need to hide. We believe that the immunoallergic component in psoriasis can be interpreted as the symbolic expression of this type of hypersensitivity.

C. THE FANTASY OF CHANGING IDENTITY

In normal human skin, as in other mammals, the cells of the corneal layer are continually shed imperceptibly and are replaced by other cells from

---

[6]In Spanish *cuero*, "leather."

deeper layers. In the psoriasis patient, cell adhesion in the corneal layer is defective and desquamation is fairly copious. This symptom can be viewed as a substitute mechanism, like the sloughing of skin in reptiles, which is a way of adapting to growth.[7] Therefore, we believe that in psoriasis an archaic behavior pattern is re-established and that both desquamation and regeneration represent a failed attempt to adapt to the demands of changes in life. In this valid recourse to a "reptile style," we also find a lack of flexibility in behavior expressed in the lack of elasticity of the skin.

In comparison to other patients with skin disorders, psoriasis patients feel more contemptible, dirty, and untouchable. They are afraid of being isolated, rejected, as if others might wish to get rid of them, and they suffer from the fantasy of being deserted. They experience exclusion as lack of recognition, in the sense of acceptance of their identity, as a rejection that places them in an inferior class, caste, or condition[8]; they feel their identity is "disgusting." The constant changes in the skin also symbolize the opposition or conflict between the purpose of changing identity, creating the illusion of the birth of a new, more accepted and valued identity on the one hand, and the illusion, on the other hand, of being inferior.[9] However, the characteristics the skin acquires in the course of the illness manifest the failure of the attempt to slough it off. Far from the longed-for recognition, there is a dramatic return of what psoriasis patients wish to repress, since they frequently inspire feelings of disgust and rejection in those who come into contact with them.

IV. The Specific Fantasy of Psoriasis— A Summary

The same unconscious emotional dispositional structure[10] produces the conscious perception of psoriasis as vasodilation and a skin infiltrate plus epidermal hyperkeratosis and parakeratosis, on the one hand, and on the other hand, the feelings represented by the expression of "being skinned

---

[7]Snakes slough all their scales after a certain time and new skin underneath is prepared to take its place. Other reptiles like lizards lose large pieces of skin in different areas. Thus, the animal temporarily becomes more sensitive to its habitat (Weisz, 1971; Viglioglia & Rubin, 1974).

[8]"Untouchable": (1) Such that it cannot or should not be touched, spoken of, or criticized; (2) applied to persons of the lowest class among the Hindus who belong to no caste and whose contact is considered dishonorable (Moliner, 1986).

[9]One of the etymologies of the term "psoriasis" is linked to the Greek *sauro*, which means lizard. This correlates with the patient's feeling of being "someone who creeps" and belongs to an "inferior order" (Korovsky, 1978).

[10]In Chapter 7, in the section "V. The Psychoanalytic View of Vascular Headaches and Cerebrovascular Accidents" on page 130 and in the section "E. Affects" on page 134, we develop the elements of psychoanalytic theory that allow us to associate somatic illness with the destructuring of the innervation keys of the affects.

alive" and "being peeled." According to our thesis, these different conscious derivatives can replace or represent each other consciously.

1. The expression "to be skinned alive" is linked directly to the somatic feeling implicit in this verbal expression. It is the feeling of being skinned alive, of having lost the protection provided by the skin organ. It refers to a feeling of being injured (and also, in an obsolete sense of the word, insulted), together with an exaggerated type of vulnerability and painful sensitivity.

Deprivation of caresses, the feeling of being in danger of losing them, or the valid absence of praise that could be fantasied as an equivalent of caresses is experienced as the presence of a bad object that injures cruelly with repeated criticism, "flaying," or skinning the subject alive. This set of feelings is the specific meaning of the particular kind of hurt feeling expressed by the term "skinned alive."

2. We think the expression "peeled" could refer to the unconscious somatic feeling of being covered with scales (which scale or peel off) that we assume to be part of mankind's phylogenetic background. Since the Spanish expression "to be scaled" refers to the suspicion aroused by an injury or trauma, the word probably refers to the fantasy of being "under cover" as the result of a traumatic experience, protecting the wound and at the same time expressing the desire to be hard and insensitive. The attempt to cover up in order to protect and conceal the injury, weakness, and hypersensitivity would be expressed by "keeping up appearances."

3. From the same unconscious emotional dispositional structure, the following meanings are structured secondarily in the conscious and are linked to the two basic fantasies of "being skinned alive" and "being peeled" that characterize psoriasis:

   a. The fantasy of growing rapidly, whose physical correlate is accelerated proliferation of immature epidermal cells.

   b. The desire and also the fear of arousing rejection by others, in order to avoid contact that might expose the patient to resentment about an early deprivation of caresses.

   c. The fantasy of changing identity and its somatic correlate: the sloughing and regeneration of the scales or patches of psoriasis, which mimic the sloughing of lizard skin, an archaic pattern inscribed in human phylogeny.

V. Case Material: Mike (Age 29)

When Mike at last decided to consult (again!) for his psoriasis, he had been shut in for two weeks in the house where he lived with his parents and sister.

   Another fit of rage . . . from head to foot! . . . as in September . . . like three and a half years ago, when he and Gabriela broke up and his psoriasis became erythrodermal.

He feels compressed, as if they had put a cast on his whole body. How can you move when you feel your skin's tight and it splits open and bleeds? Immobile inside the pajama soaked in the disgusting car oil they recommended, he thinks: I'll have to wait . . . it's happened before. He knows he'll lose all his skin, that his nails will fall off and then grow in again, that the sheets will be covered with scales and that, finally, he'll be able to move again. . . .

But in the meantime, who knows what messes they'll be making in the factory. . . . Dad and Morris . . . that old fogy who'd never have been their partner if he hadn't put up the money. When they argued over the boiler last month, Morris was forced to admit he was right . . . but they always argued. . . .

Mike thinks that if the factory is doing well, it's because he built it up from nothing and does his all to keep it going. The only thing they do is scathe him . . . and shame him in front of the employees!

But they're not going to see him go down . . . they never saw him weak even when he was little, when he wished so much his mother would pat his head or his back. Mamma! always so docile and good-natured . . . but so lost in her own world . . . she had to be taken care of . . .

He would have liked to feel Dad's hand on his shoulder, like a friend's . . . you can't fix anything up with expensive presents . . . if only he'd hit him! . . . Once, he felt the sting of his hand on his face! Once . . . because he was naughty, he hit him and was sorry right away.

Gabriela, his first and only love, was always distant. . . . Of course: she had to put up with the psoriasis! In spite of that, she really loved him . . . he thinks he can't be wrong about that. . . . Then, she left him, when everything had gone bad, the marijuana, the Thalassa,[11] and the alcohol.

The other women (how many were there?) he had involved himself with only in an attempt to forget her, but he never, ever, fell in love again! Now, all that was left was sex. Now, he doesn't dare to think of tenderness or caresses . . . the fear they might hurt him torments him. . . . Only alcohol makes it a little better. . . . There's something, Mike thinks, that's eating at his soul: he can't even remember the name of the last woman he slept with!

His only solace is his pride in what he made of the factory . . . but now they criticize him! . . . Dad and Morris . . . they don't praise him anymore, like they used to. . . . Sometimes, he'd like to go and hide away . . . somewhere . . . but they'd better not imagine they're going to see him go down! . . . If it weren't for the psoriasis . . . they wouldn't be able to irritate him (*sic!*), he'd walk all over all of them. . . .

It started when he was fourteen . . . on his head, back, and elbows . . . in Brazil, where they had gone to live because of Dad's business. In

---

[11]A codeine-containing cough medicine which the patient abused.

Brazil . . . alone and far away . . . where Mom had gone crazy . . . he felt so scared when she heard voices and had those epileptic fits . . . and so ashamed . . . there, he had to grow up all of a sudden. . . . Finally, there was no choice but to return . . . and Dad, who couldn't get used to it, stopped working.

All the money they'd been able to accumulate had to be spent on doctors! . . . because Mom, who got worse, didn't leave the house for six months . . . and he, in the meantime, did nothing but eat. . . . He put on 73 pounds!

He couldn't get up the courage to study medicine, like Dad wanted him to, so he started to study to be a veterinarian, but he gave that up too. . . . Until Gabriela came along, nothing had come out right . . . except the diet . . . with which, in six months, all of a sudden, he had gotten the fat off.

Everything had gotten more and more difficult. . . . Gabriela wanted something more . . . and the psoriasis that couldn't be quenched! . . . When she left, the marijuana wasn't enough anymore. The Thalassa and the tranquilizers didn't help him either . . . the nightmare of the nights, shut inside, smoking with friends, in the dining room where he slept . . . it got dirtier and dirtier . . . he didn't want them to see it like that . . . under fire from the damned illness . . . that advanced, for the first time, to the point that it covered his whole body. . . .

He couldn't stand to see himself like that . . . he couldn't stand it now either, three years later . . . and he asked Morris to find him an apartment where he could live alone . . . far from his parents' house . . . hadn't he paid for his drug addiction by working unflinchingly? . . .

But living alone! . . . without anybody to help him. . . .

When he was seven and his sister Adela was born, he would sometimes choke with fits of asthma . . . and he got so scared . . . and then it was even worse, when her lungs got sick before she was a year old and they had to hospitalize her for six months with Mom. . . . Six months (!) when nobody remembered he existed. . . .

Would he be tough[12] enough to face up to it now . . . to live alone? . . .

He had so much wished his mother would pat his head or his back, when he was little. His father hadn't realized how much Mike "hungered" for caresses either. The bronchial asthma of infancy, worsening when he was eight because of his little sister's six-month-long hospitalization, evidences a deep crisis in an intensely dependent relationship with his mother.

In puberty, the asthma went away, and then it happened that Mom, ever more lost in her world, suddenly disappeared in her episode of

---

[12]The idiomatic expression in Spanish for "being tough enough for something" can be translated literally as "to have enough leather for. . . ."

madness. Mike prefers to feel that his mother is docile and good-natured, but she is a mother who, in spite of the fear and shame she causes him, had to be cared for . . . because Dad, who couldn't get used to it, couldn't manage. The anger, the resentment, and the feeling of injustice in the face of what he experienced as another, unbearable desertion, disappear from consciousness and he has his first outbreak of psoriasis.

This medium-intensity psoriasis reveals his need to grow up fast in order to take care of his family like a man and at the same time to create a "protective shell" for himself to defend him from the wound left by the constant threat of another desertion. It was an attempt to show he was strong by appearing to have a "thick skin" when he was feeling that he wasn't "tough enough" to take care of his mother.

Gabriela's desertion left him "skinned alive," and his psoriasis spread and became erythrodermal. He would have liked to appear hard and insensitive, but he felt more hurt than ever. It was a desperate attempt to trust in someone, and it failed, which made him feel even more "scaled," in the sense of having been swindled or having learned the hard way, and also of feeling hardened. Along with this, his illness leads him to succumb to the unconscious temptation to block his illusions of love and arouse the rejection he feared from the outset.

In the following three years, he began to work as a man does, and when he began to feel that the praise satisfied his hunger for caresses, when he began to "be somebody," his father and Morris began to criticize him, irritating him and again "skinning him alive." Perhaps the time had come for him to look for a place of his own, somewhere he could "be a new man," but he needs the reassurance that someone will take care of him, because he is not aware of the fact that precisely because he's scaled, he is not tough enough, even if he won't give in[13] in his attempts to get ahead.

---

[13]The expression in Spanish is *d Flojarle*, meaning literally "let things go loose," "to become lax."

3

THE MEANINGS OF RESPIRATION

L. A. Chiozza, O. Baldino,
M. Funosas, E. Obstfeld

> If we may rely upon the evidence of
> language, it was movement of the air that
> provided the prototype of intellectuality
> [Geistigkeit], for intellect [Geist] derives
> its name from a breath of wind—animus,
> spiritus, and the Hebrew *ruach* (breath).
> This too led to the discovery of the mind
> [Seele (soul)] as that of the intellectual
> [geistigen] principle in individual human
> beings. Observation found the movement
> of air once again in men's breathing,
> which ceases when they die. To this day a
> dying man "breathes out his spirit"
> [Seele]. Now, however, the world of
> spirits [Geisterreich] lay open to men.
> [Freud, 1939a, p. 114]

I. Introduction

We base our theories on an epistemological conception that allows us to
affirm that the categories we call "soma" and "psyche" result from the
fact that knowledge is structured around two conceptual organizations:
one is "physical" and the other "historical" (Chiozza, 1972, 1976, 1986).
The former, the origin of the natural sciences, includes all that we perceive as physical form, function, disturbance, evolution, or development.
The latter, the foundation of the sciences whose object is culture, refers
to a register which is experienced as a certain fantasy or as a meaning,
inherent in a particular material existence.

25

Both organizations, neither reducible to the other, derive from the same unconscious existence, which is in itself neither psychical nor somatic. This unconscious source is sometimes expressed through what is consciously perceived as a transformation of the physical organ, sometimes through what consciousness interprets as the meaning of an emotional state. This source is what we consciously call a specific unconscious fantasy; we represent it as a scene related to acts (Freud & Breuer, 1895d) and functions that were originally appropriate and full of meaning. Organic functioning as well as the uses of language and myth are derivatives or partial aspects of the specific unconscious fantasy.

The respiratory representations that we have found in biology, literature, myths, common language, and etymology furnish us with a broader understanding of the meanings of breathing. In the next section of this chapter, we discuss the importance of oxygen for life and in the third, the importance of the respiratory function of oxygen transport. In Section IV, "Respiration as a symbol," we develop ideas taken from literature, myths, and common language. In the following section, we discuss our thesis on the specific affects linked to the metabolic and pulmonary respiratory functions, following the psychoanalytic theory of the affects. In Section VI, we describe the vicissitudes of the affect of "discouragement" that is specific to both normal and pathological aspects of pulmonary respiration. Section VII summarizes the concepts discussed, and the next reviews the ideas of several psychoanalysts regarding asthma, as well as those we have discussed in this paper. The last section illustrates the theory with the cases of three patients suffering from bronchial asthma: one without complications, another with chronic obstructive bronchiopulmonary disease and a third with recurrent pneumonia.

II. Oxygen and Life

The high proportion of oxygen among the elements forming protoplasm and its role as an agent of combustion in all vital phenomena indicate that it is a basic element of life. The creatures called anaerobes are those that are unable to live in free oxygen. Absolute anaerobes can live only by using the oxygen bound to decomposing organic or mineral substances. The property of being able to live deprived of free oxygen is observed in tiny bacteria or in organisms that have not evolved to the level of significant cellular differentiation. In superior organisms, aerobic life includes the property of using the combined oxygen that is always involved in their biochemical activities.

Biological experimentation shows that the level of cellular activity is determined by the relationship between oxygen demand and supply, and that death takes place when oxygen no longer participates in biochemical reactions (Morales Macedo, 1955).

A portion of the oxygen provided by plants is converted into ozone (O_3) in the upper atmosphere through the action of the ultraviolet radiation originating in the sun. This layer of ozone filters the bands of ultraviolet light that are most damaging to nucleic acids and proteins while allowing the visible light necessary for photosynthesis to pass through. Without this semipermeability, human life would never have come into existence (Hoyle & Wickramasinghe, 1978; Thomas, 1974).

> One could say that the advent of oxygen into the atmosphere was the result of evolution or on the contrary that evolution sprang from the advent of oxygen. It is the same. Once the photosynthetic cells appeared . . . the future respiratory mechanism of the Earth was set up. . . . When anaerobic life was threatened (by the increase in oxygen in the atmosphere), the inevitable solution was the advent of mutants with oxidation systems and ATP (adenosine triphosphate). With this, an explosive stage of development began in which great varieties of aerobic life became possible, including the multi-cellular forms. [Thomas, 1974, p. 223]

Something like this is to be found in J. E. Lovelock's "Gaia hypothesis" (1979). He declared that

> the physical and chemical conditions of the Earth's surface, the atmosphere and the oceans, have been and are adequate for life thanks to the very presence of life, which contrasts with conventional wisdom according to which life and planetary conditions followed separate paths, the former adapting to the latter. [Lovelock, 1979, p. 178]

Lungs, i.e., organs allowing direct exchange of gases with the environment, developed in the last stage of the evolution of animal species (reptiles, birds, and mammals), when water was no longer the only natural environment for life. This exchange of gases is effected by diffusion through the point of contact between the blood and the environment, i.e., the alveolocapillary membrane. Since oxygen diffuses through a membrane, it could be said that the quantity of the gas that passes through the membrane depends on the pressure, thickness, and nature of the membrane, and especially on the area of the contact surface.

Animals' need for oxygen varies widely. Any activity involving expenditure of energy increases oxygen consumption. This happens, for example, when metabolism is intensified as a consequence of physical exercise or of digestion or fever. Whereas lower animals need little oxygen and apparently cannot regulate its consumption and aquatic animals do so only indirectly (by seeking oxygen-rich water), vertebrates can generally adapt automatically to variable needs by modifying the frequency and amplitude of respiratory movements (Vogel & Angerman, 1974). Therefore, we may conjecture that the (motor) action leading to increased oxygenation—configured phylogenetically as an appropriate motor act[1]—was related to an increase in activity that created a need for adaptation. We shall return to this idea later.

The energy that organisms require for maintenance of vital functions and for action in the external world derives from the oxidation of food products. The global chemical result of these processes of oxidation is constant oxygen consumption and the production of carbon dioxide and water, plus other residual products of lesser quantitative importance, such as sulfates and diverse nitrogenated compounds.

Nearly all the substances oxidized in the tissues are not affected by oxygen when outside the tissues at physiological temperatures and pH. They are easily oxidized within the organism as a result of the catalytic action of enzymes which accelerate certain stages of the process. Many cellular oxidation processes occur with a decrease in the free energy of the system. This decrease represents the maximum useful work that can be obtained from them. Organisms also have mechanisms that enable the storage and use of oxygen for the many functions indispensable for normal life.

The use of the energy provided by oxidation is not direct but takes place through special mechanisms. The most important of these is the synthesis of phosphorus complexes, forming the "phosphoryl groups" (e.g., adenosine triphosphate, or ATP) with high energy content. The energy that can be stored in these groups forms the real energy reserve provided by oxidation.

III. Respiratory Function

In unicellular organisms gas exchange occurs directly between the cell and its environment, whereas in multicellular organisms this process is mediated by the respiratory and circulatory systems.

Phylogenetic development of new life forms involved a greater need for oxygenation. The passage from aquatic life to land life allowed the

---

[1]Freud stated that a hysterical attack is a motor act appropriate for the traumatic scene in childhood. "Appropriate" or "expedient" in this context means "having a meaning in the interior of a psychical series" (cf. his *Psychopathology of Everyday Life* [1901b]). Later, he maintained that the affects were equivalent to universal, congenital hysterical attacks (cf. his "Inhibitions, symptoms, anxiety" [1926d]), so that the affects may be considered motor acts which at one time in phylogeny were appropriate. Thus, he stated that "In order to understand a hysterical attack, all one has to do is to look for the situation in which the movements in question formed part of an appropriate and expedient action" (Freud, 1926d, p. 134). Elsewhere, he wrote, "To make myself more intelligible—an affective state would be constructed in the same way as a hysterical attack and, like it, would be the precipitate of a reminiscence. A hysterical attack may thus be likened to a freshly constructed individual affect, and a normal affect to the expression of a general hysteria which has become a heritage" (Freud, 1916–1917, p. 396).

swim bladder of the fish to develop into the lungs of the amphibians, reptiles, birds, and mammals. The increase in respiratory capacity was achieved not by a great increase in size but by a subdivision of the lungs into smaller and smaller sacs. Thus, the structure of the lungs became increasingly complex as the need for oxygenation grew. The configuration of the alveolar sacs increased the respiratory surface; at the same time, the respiratory mechanism led to increase in variations of amplitude and frequency, thus also actively influencing the magnitude of gas exchange.

During inhalation in human beings muscular action lowers the diaphragm and raises the ribs, widening the chest. Atmospheric pressure then pushes air into the widened chest cavity. During exhalation, the muscles rest, the chest narrows, and air is expelled. This combined rhythmic action takes place around sixteen times a minute when the subject is resting. Frequency is controlled mainly by the respiratory center in the medulla, which responds to changes in the level of hydrogen and carbon dioxide ions in the blood, as well as other factors such as changes in temperature, motor activities, and neurovegetative alterations.

Oxygen, diffused through the capillary membranes of the network surrounding the alveoli, combines with hemoglobin in the red corpuscles. This oxygenated blood, pumped by the heart, reaches the tissues by way of the arterial network.

Carbon dioxide takes the reverse path, circulating in the blood as a bicarbonate ion, combined with hemoglobin, and as a dissolved gas. Only in the third form is it available for diffusion in the lungs and exhalation.

The lungs of the fetus are not used for gas exchange; before birth they have a secretory function and are one of the main sources of amniotic fluid (Murray, 1983). The glucose reserves in the lungs, which increase until gestation is nearly at its end and then decrease, are probably a reservoir for the carbohydrates required by the pulmonary cells to satisfy their energy needs and also by the rest of the growing organism. The lungs are also the production site for surfactant effects[2] necessary for ventilatory function, which begins with the first postnatal respiration and continues throughout life.

Fetal development takes place in a very protected medium: aquatic, hypoxic, and acidemic, in contrast to that in which extrauterine life develops. In order to ensure survival in the very different extrauterine medium, adaptations must take place rapidly after delivery. In the few minutes the placenta requires to separate from the uterus, the newborn must activate the central and autonomic nervous systems, replace the liquid filling the lungs with air, establish the pulmonary circulation,

---

[2]The alveoli are lined with a thin liquid layer of lipoproteins, phospholipids with surfactant effects, whose decrease favors collapse, e.g., in atelectasia.

and reorganize the direction of blood flow through the cardiac chambers and the main blood vessels. These processes are not separate but rather interdependent phenomena essential for the development of a cardiorespiratory system capable of maintaining an adequate supply of oxygen.

The culmination of delivery is the first breath; this event is considered the end of fetal existence and the beginning of postnatal life. But before this, the respiratory center of the central nervous system must integrate the afferent impulses that reach it and initiate efferent signals to the muscles of respiration (Murray, 1983). The fact that the fetus's respiratory gas exchange is accomplished in the placenta—whose oxygen supply is constant—defines one aspect of the fetus's dependency on the mother. With the initiation of postnatal life and rhythmic pulmonary respiration, the individual receives the direct supply of oxygen that allows independence. One of the significant differences between prenatal and postnatal respiration is linked to the fact that the former is peremptory while the latter is capable of waiting, an aspect we will discuss below.

IV. RESPIRATION AS A SYMBOL

A. RESPIRATION AS THE SYMBOL FOR THE SOUL AND THE SPIRIT

A relation between respiration and all that is spiritual can be traced to classical antiquity and is seen in literature and mythology, as well as in etymology or ordinary language. In Greek philosophy, air was considered the principle of life (Anaximenes, in Ferrater Mora, 1954). "Air" or "pneuma" has meant simply the essential element constituting each thing or even the "divine breath," the representation of the Holy Spirit, the creator and regulator of the world (Ferrater Mora, 1954).

The Bible states that "then the Lord God formed man of dust from the ground, and breathed into his nostrils the breath of life; and man became a living being" (Genesis 2.7). A Pelasgian myth narrates the union between the goddess Eurynome and the air, embodied by her in the serpent Orphion and describes how the universe was born of this union (Victor Civita Editor, 1973). A Greek myth tells the story of the love of Psyche and Eros for one another. According to Perez Rioja (1962), "Psyche is the personification of the human soul, the object loved by Eros." Psyche is also the symbol of spirituality. She is usually represented as a beautiful young woman with butterfly's wings. "Psyche" means "soul" and also "air," "breath," "living being," "life," and "spirit."

A Polynesian creation myth presents an impersonal being called "Io" which creates the cosmic substance with a breath. Io is considered the soul of the world and therefore both subject and object of creation (Grimal, 1963). Brahman mythology also relates air to spirit and creation. For the Hindus, the life-giving properties of respiration extend to universal creation. In religious rituals, the repetition of the Sanskrit word "Om" evokes the act by which Brahma created the world: it is a long expiration with which the inner being participates in the forces of the universe (Eliade, 1955, 1964).

Spanish includes many words whose etymological root comes from the Latin verb *spirare*, which means "to blow" and "to breathe." Among these we find: "spirit," "inspire," "aspire," "expire," "respiration," "sigh," and "perspire." Another series of terms in Spanish is derived from the Latin *anhelare* (to breathe with difficulty) such as "breath encouragement," "to encourage," and "to yearn for" = "to desire." On the other hand, "exhale" derives from the Latin *exhalare*, which means "to make gases, vapors, or odors go out," related to breath, vapor, respiration, and *halare*, which means "to sigh or to whimper" (Moliner, 1986).

According to Barcia (1961), the Spanish word for "sighing," *suspirar*, is composed of "sub" (under) and "spirit," conveying the idea of a respiration that comes from the depths of the soul, a deep and difficult breath but not relating to a painful situation, since we often sigh over a happy event, as if to bid past anxieties farewell. After an affliction we may sigh, and the sigh in this situation is not a sign of grief but of relief. To sigh is to open the chest, to breathe deeply: it implies a previous oppression. Therefore, the sigh is preceded by a situation in which "breath was cut off"; it is a heavy and prolonged inspiration followed by an equally long expiration, its special and audible representative. It is a "respiration" that comes from the depths of the soul, as the etymology of the Spanish word shows. Sighing comes after a brief moment of breathlessness, a brief strangling or choking, as it were, so that the expiration in sighing (in Spanish *desahogo*, literally, dechoking[3]) is a recovery from lack of breath/ discouragement.

In ordinary language we find several expressions linked to air, such as: "to put on airs" (to give oneself importance), "to have an air" (to look like), "to get the air" (to be rejected), "to breeze through" (to get over a difficulty successfully or easily), "to be up in the air" (to be undecided or out of touch with reality). The person who breezes through feels "light" in the sense of feeling spiritually satisfied at having overcome that difficulty, which is symbolized by breathing easily. The exclamation "oof!," signifying irritation, fatigue, or suffocation, is associated with the idea of blowing out or swelling up, of mockery or scorn. The sound evokes the sudden escape of pent-up air, as when a person "blows up," expressing violent anger. This expression represents an intense and peremptory attempt to "let off steam." When something spiritual is evident in what concerns everybody, we tend to speak of spirit,

---

[3]*Desahogo* also means "to give vent to one's feelings," "to get something off one's chest."

as in the case of expressions that refer to the spirit of a group ("esprit de corps"), a society, a people, or an epoch. From this point of view, spirit can be considered to be "in" the individuals or "among" them, the collective form of the psyche.

Wyss (1947) affirmed that the air we breathe, the "pneuma" or "breath of life," was used as a symbol of the spirit, which is the principle of constant renewal of our inner life and with which we have a reciprocal relationship. He added that the word needs the respiratory organs in order to be spoken; he concluded that the respiratory organs are not only means for renewing our vital energy but also for spiritualizing life. In Wyss' opinion, respiration is the first (postnatal) experience of our link with the external world as well as the first experience of an external resistance. It is the first postnatal communication that we establish with our environment, a communication that is involuntarily and rhythmically verified under the command of an urgent need.[4]

Weizsaecker (1950b) stated that respiration implies a relationship with a substance in the environment in the form of a gas, that is, the air (oxygen), and that this relationship involves an exchange that takes place through a rhythmic function. When this activity of entry and exit, of inspiration and expiration, is altered, as in the case of dyspnea, death anxiety is evoked. This anxiety, which emerges rapidly and is intense, is kept at abeyance only through that same rhythmic respiratory activity.

The respiratory function is peremptory: it can be interrupted voluntarily for a short time, but involuntary control appears and respiration is then re-established automatically.[5] That peremptoriness is greater than that of other functions and makes respiration especially appropriate for symbolizing relationships in which there are strong feelings of dependency.

From a symbolic perspective, the spirit that unites us all is represented by air, since this element is shared by all. The relationship with air is the specific symbol for living together. Appropriate social exchange, implying the experience of a good relationship with others, can be symbolized by the efficient action of harmonious respiration, of a rhythmic movement between inspiration and expiration (Obstfeld et al., 1975, 1983a, 1983b).

Obstfeld et al. (1975) pointed out that pulmonary function, implying sharing something in common (air), is connected to the capacity for

---

[4]The respiratory tract is also the entryway for pathogenic germs, which are, in a figurative sense, the enemy forces we have to confront in our relationship with the external world (Wyss, 1947).

[5]Wyss (1947) declared that the voluntary innervation of the respiratory system for the most part serves audible language. It is possible to think that through audible language we attempt to reestablish the original union that was lost. Physiology teaches that during phonation sensitivity to CO_2 decreases notably and the subject withstands levels of arterial pCO_2 considerably higher than those tolerated when it is inactive (Murray, 1983).

empathy and the desire for deep understanding. They found that some famous personalities who had pulmonary disorders (Dostoievsky, Bolivar, Schreber, "Che" Guevara) experienced similar situations: the difficulty of realizing a social ideal.

In other words: normal respiratory function, implying the exchange of gases with the environment, symbolizes adequate social and spiritual exchange with the objects in the surroundings. For this reason, the word "atmosphere" is used to refer to the shared portion of both air and society.

B. Creation and Respiration

It is meaningful that the word "inspiration" designates not only part of the respiratory process, the inhalation of air, but also the "effect the writer, orator or artist feels, the singular and effective stimulation that makes him or her produce something spontaneously, as if it had been found suddenly and not sought for with effort" (Real Academia Española, 1950). Etymologically, "inspire," deriving from the Latin *spirare*, means "to breathe into," "to infuse ideas" (Corominas, 1961).

Pulmonary inspiration symbolizes the inspiration that stimulates creation. This is evidenced by the use of the same word to represent both processes and the fact that in both myth and literature, the act of creation is represented by the involvement of air, wind, or a "stimulating breath" by which matter is animated.

The fact that the same word denotes two different events—the physiological phenomenon and the creative state of mind—allows us to think that they share a common nucleus of unconscious meaning and that these events are therefore linked to each other by a specific relationship. Inspiration, as a momentary event of the respiratory process, incorporates the air that is indispensable for the maintenance of life (*zoe*) and also, as a moment of the creative process, it keeps spiritual development (*bios*) alive.[6] In the figurative sense "inspire" refers to the act by which God illuminates understanding or excites and moves the will, and in mystical theology, the "soul's burning affect for God" is "aspiration" (Real Academia Española, 1950).

When Octavio Paz (1956) discussed poetic inspiration, he maintained that the poet's voice is, and is not, his own. The one who makes him say things he did not mean to say is called "daimon," "muse,"

---

[6]Inspiration was classically considered to be a power which, coming from outside, illuminated the artist. For Plato, the poet is possessed; his delusion and enthusiasm are signs of demonic possession. Dante tells us that in dreams, Love dictates and inspires his poems, like a revelation involving superior powers (Paz, 1956). Greek mythology associates inspiration allegorically with a flaming altar, with the horse Pegasus, and with the color yellow (Perez Rioja, 1962). Pegasus is the winged horse of the Muses that symbolizes "the ascendant power of elevation, thanks to the innate capacity for spiritualization." The nine Muses were the inspirers and protectresses of the arts and sciences.

"spirit," "genius," "work," "chance," "unconscious," or "reason."[7] He held that inspiration is nothing and is nowhere. It is only aspiration, a going, a moving forward, toward what we ourselves are: an exercise in liberty and transcendency. Only after the world has been emptied of meaning can the poet leap to found a new meaning and invent another world: the poetic world. Through inspiration, man realizes himself, becomes "another." It is when he takes this big leap that tears him away from himself that he can give himself up and be "lost" in the other (Paz, 1956).

These reflections, referring to the art of poetry, can be extended to every human activity involving a creative process. Personal and social life require this "inspiration," thanks to which the exit from enclosure and the approach to "the other" enable access to a new reality, product of a re-creation. In this sense, it is difficult for inspiration to thrust us beyond ourselves when the prevailing desire is to remain in a confined and isolated world without ecosystemic connection.

From the psychoanalytic point of view, we can think of inspiration as a moment of increased permeability of the id, the source of universal unconscious meanings. Pulmonary inspiration predominantly denotes the entry of air into the lungs; aspiration, as a physical process, on the other hand, predominantly denotes the act by which air is removed from a certain place. Creative inspiration accompanies the act of creation of a work; aspiration, as an experience, accompanies a desire that has not been realized. Whereas the cigarette smoker places the accent on the inspiration of the smoke, the pipe smoker places it on the aspiration. One might say that the former represents the difficulty of "being inspired" whereas for the latter this symptomatic act is a substitute for the aspirations that he is unable to reach.

The close ties between inspiration and respiration lead us to conclude that, just as repression of the failure of the capacity to materialize projects can be expressed specifically in a liver disorder (Chiozza, 1963), repression of the awareness of the absence of creative inspiration could become manifest, also in a specific way, as a respiratory disorder.

C. SYMBIOSIS AND RESPIRATION

Studies of hepatic fantasies (Chiozza, 1963, 1974a, 1984) led us to think that specific unconscious fantasies of respiration and oral fantasies are

---

[7]In order to understand the essence of inspiration, the author first introduces his conception of mankind. Mankind is not something made, finished, but something that is always in the process of being made, although this implies neither that mankind is taking something from within nor receiving it from without. In that constant activity of creating itself, mankind is like an arrow shot into the air, skimming the air and falling beyond itself, at each step being an "other" as well as itself. As for Man's "otherness," it is in each of us, and when the poet creates, he or she leaves him/herself, only to be him/herself (Paz, 1956). We also find the word "aspiration" linked to the inspiration of respiratory physiology. It receives the representation of the desire, longing, or impulse to achieve something, as can be seen in the use of the same word for both processes.

contained in a more regressive form in hepatic fantasies. During the period of gestation, nourishment and oxygen reach the fetus through the mother's placenta. Later, as a consequence of birth, mother and child become "independent" of each other; at the same time, the respiratory and digestive functions are differentiated. The child no longer uses the mother for breathing and takes up this function autonomously. Postnatal respiration can therefore be said to symbolize the break-up of maternal-filial symbiosis and the initiation of a new order of dependency.

Freud (1916–1917) stated that the model for anxiety is the act of birth. In the same text, Freud explained that the word "anxiety" (*Angst*, which also means "narrowing") stresses the characteristic of lack of breath, which as a consequence of a real situation at birth, is often reproduced later in affects. Freud affirmed that the first state of anxiety originates in the separation of the fetus from the mother. In clinical practice, we observe that the difficulties patients experience when undergoing situations of change whose characteristics evoke the birth trauma are frequently expressed by respiratory disorders.

V. The Effective Action and the Affects Involved in Respiration

A. The Affects in Psychoanalytic Theory

An affect is a process that shares the characteristics of the sign and the symbol. As an indicator of presence (sign), it is part of a "real" somatic event that expresses a current motor discharge affecting the ego (Freud, 1915e). As a representative of absence (symbol), it constitutes an "ideal" psychical phenomenon, a "memorial monument" referring to an unconscious reminiscence (Freud & Breuer, 1895d; Chiozza, 1986a). It is like a universal, congenital hysterical attack that represents a motor event that was appropriate in an earlier stage of phylogeny.

In psychoanalytic theory, the affect is "psychosomatic" par excellence, since this concept offers the advantage of being relevant to both categories (reminiscence and current discharge), thus eliminating the traditional split between psyche and soma (Chiozza, 1986a). The affect is thus perceived on the one hand as a current physical event and on the other as a psychical, historical event whose meaning can be interpreted.

In metapsychological terms, the affect is a vegetative motor discharge whose magnitude forms a complementary series with the quota of motor discharge involved in the action exerted on the materially present object. Each affect is a vegetative movement carried out in a characteristic way (whose "ultimate consequences" are perceived by the conscious mind in a series that ranges from "somatic" sensations to sentiments). Discharges of this type are determined by an unconscious mnemic trace from an earlier stage of phylogeny conveyed by a customary "record" that Freud (1900a) called the "innervation key,"[8] an idea that we attribute to what he called the "unrepressed unconscious" (Freud, 1915b). As a result of repeated elaborations on this subject (Chiozza, 1976), we concluded that from the metapsychological perspective, "somatic" illness implies that the displacement of the cathexis does not operate as in neurosis on a substitute representation but "within" the innervation key of the affects, so that some elements of the key receive a more intense cathexis than others. In this sense, all somatic illnesses can be conceived of as the "decomposition" of the innervation key of an affect during its discharge.

B. THE AFFECTS CONNECTED WITH THE RESPIRATORY FUNCTION

We will attempt to characterize the affects relating to respiratory function in order to deepen our understanding of its specific unconscious meaning. The term "spirits" denotes a general state that as a basic disposition, temperament, or mood colors the activities of life and alludes to our attitude toward action: "spirited" or "dispirited." This disposition for action that we call spirit and the energy derived from metabolic processes (according to medical knowledge) are expressions—which the conscious mind categorizes as psychical and somatic, respectively—of a single unconscious fantasy, the same entity, a single structural matrix, that constitutes their source.

In Spanish, the word *aliento*, which comes from the Latin *anhelitare* (Corominas, 1961), in the sense of "encourage," refers basically to the air we breathe. The verb *alentar* means first to breathe, to take in, and to release air with the lungs. Its meaning in the figurative sense alludes to the building up of our own hope, love, or hate. It also refers to the action

---

[8]For Freud affects do not exist in the unconscious as present "actualities"; instead, dispositions to the development of a given affect are present there (cf. Freud [1915e], "The unconscious"). The type of disposition in question is an unconscious idea, an unconscious representation. Freud made it clear (cf. Freud [1900a], *The Interpretation of Dreams*, p. 582) that the idea is a *code* or *key* that determines the innervations that constitute the different somatic discharges typical of each affect. Somatic phenomena such as mydriasis or tachycardia, for example, are the product of innervations that are part of the key of the fear-affect. This is so in physiological conditions. When the affect is repressed and the whole cathexis moves to one of the elements of the innervation key, we find a pathophysiologic state, for example, paroxysmal tachycardia, which is a pathosomatic deformation, a somatic equivalent of the fear-affect—that is, a pathosomatic deformation of the innervation key (cf. Chiozza [1974], *La transformaciòn del afecto en languaje*).

Affective states have become incorporated in the mind as precipitates of primaeval traumatic experiences, and when a similar situation occurs they are revived like mnemic symbols. I do not think I have been wrong in likening them to the more recent and individually acquired hysterical attack and in regarding them as its normal prototypes [Freud, 1926d, p. 93].

. . . I should be inclined to regard them [affective states] as universal, typical and innate hysterical attacks, as compared to the recently and individually acquired attacks which occur in hysterical neuroses and whose origin and significance as mnemic symbols have been revealed by analysis [Freud, 1926d, p. 133].

of giving a person spirit, of encouraging the person to realize a certain action (Moliner, 1986). In this sense, the person who is encouraged acquires "vigorous animation, strength or courage" (Real Academia Española, 1950). The word "breath" also refers to being alive, for example, in the expression "to one's last breath," which means "until one's last moment of life."

In the case of pulmonary respiration, from a shared unconscious matrix the sensations and perceptions corresponding to breath as the product of pulmonary respiration reach the conscious system, along with the particular experience of receiving encouragement that is implicit in the meaning of the verb "to animate." For this reason, pulmonary respiration can be assigned the representation of "breath/encouragement" and of the affective state corresponding to being "encouraged."

While being encouraged and animated are unconscious, discouragement and dispiritedness are typical and universal affects which frequently reach consciousness and acquire the category of feelings. These feelings are given the names of "discouragement" and "dispiritedness" precisely because the disorders that lead to what the conscious categorizes as lack of air or of energy are assigned the representation of the complete affective process, since the unconscious structural matrix of the respiratory function of the lungs and metabolism configures a part of the innervation key of that affective process.

VI. Discouragement and Pulmonary Respiration

A. On the Innervation Key of Discouragement and Dispiritedness

In an earlier report (Chiozza, 1981) we discussed the distinction between diverse clinical forms of melancholia, some of them characterized as digestive, hepatic, or cardiac, depending on the predominance in them of sourness, bitterness, or nostalgia. We can likewise refer to a "respiratory" form of melancholia, characterized essentially by discouragement.

The most characteristic mood of what in psychiatric clinical practice is called "depression" seems to be discouragement. However, according to what we have said, discouragement is a particular form of lack of spirit and often takes over its representation. Noyes (1951) and Ey et al. (1965) describe reduction in basal metabolism in depression. Dumas (1933), basing his thesis on the laboratory experiments of Badonnel, affirmed that such lowering of the metabolic rate is a global expression of the decrease in oxidation that takes place in most tissues. He maintained that the rhythm of respiration is diminished and that respiration itself becomes superficial and is interrupted by long pauses. We can infer that variations in metabolic energetic processes are what are felt, in the realm of experience, as variations in mood, and that both phenomena derive from the same unconscious key. The affects of discouragement and lack of spirit can be compared to minor forms of melancholic depression. From this perspective, we can safely suppose that many of the somatic alterations described in depression are "innervations" belonging to the "key" that corresponds to these affects. Unfortunately, psychiatric descriptions help little, since they describe too many different signs and symptoms without order or coherence.[9]

We must be satisfied for now with the hypothesis that the metabolic respiratory function, in the case of dispiritedness, and the pulmonary respiratory function, in the case of discouragement, are the prime elements in the respective innervation keys of these affects.

B. HIBERNATION: A PHYSIOLOGICAL REACTION RELATED TO DISCOURAGEMENT AND DISPIRITEDNESS

Biology describes a model of adaptive defense called "hibernation." When an animal hibernates, it reduces its metabolism to a minimum, body temperature drops, respiration is nearly null, and it falls into a kind of lethargy that enables it to subsist in hostile environments. Hibernation implies that the animal has adopted a form of isolation from its surroundings and is awaiting an improvement in environmental conditions. In hibernation, then, one may hypothesize that the body functions that "languish"[10] constitute an adaptation favoring survival in a food-scarce environment. The

---

[9]Henry Ey found digestive disturbances (anorexia, nausea, constipation, or diarrhea, hepatobiliary disorders); cardiovascular disorders (alteration of the pulse and arterial pressure); amenorrhea; and muscular hypotonia and hypostesia in depressed patients. Noyes (1951), Darwin (1872), and Dumas (1933) coincide in their description of characteristic gestures of what Noyes calls "depression"; for Darwin these are the expression of "dejection," "anguish," "grief," "discouragement," or "despair," and for Dumas they are manifestations of "passive sadness." They observe that circulation languishes, the face grows pale and drawn, the muscles dilate, the eyelids lower, the head drops to the oppressed chest; the lips, cheeks, and lower jaw fall; and the eyes are inexpressive, wide open, and staring and lose their shine, sometimes with tears in them. The eyebrows are oblique (the inner corner is raised); the forehead wrinkles, the corners of the mouth turn down, and the lines between nose and lips deepen. Dumas also noted that in sadness the color of the skin and hair changes. The skin looks purplish and sometimes white; some people have a pale face and the brachial and crural extremities are bluish. This is due to the slackening of the peripheral circulation. The hair loses its shine as a result of decrease in sebaceous secretion and also in its nutrition. The authors describe other signs like sleep disturbances, altered sexual appetite, inhibition of thought and psychomotor activity, slowness in initiation and execution, slow respiration, with sighs and the "need to receive encouragement in order to eat," as if they felt they were unworthy of receiving food.

According to Dumas, the most intense feelings in passive sadness are of powerlessness and discouragement; the whole body experiences sadness: the head drops, the legs fold, the arms hang down, the entire organism loses control. The patients feel the rhythm of their movements is diminished; they can barely get warm, their hands are cold, they shiver (chapter IV, p. 446). Although Dumas described various depressive feelings in passive sadness, he stated that the content of the affective state of "sadness" goes beyond the description of weakness, discouragement, resignation, and organic and mental slackening. He believes that all those affective states may be components of sadness, but that they do not in themselves constitute it. The feeling of sadness may reach consciousness without resignation, powerlessness, or discouragement and yet still persist. Further, physical and mental powerlessness and discouragement may be conscious while sadness is not felt.

[10]"Languish": to be or become feeble, weak, or enervated; to be, or live, in a state of depression or decreasing vitality; to become dispirited; to suffer neglect (*Merriam-Webster's Dictionary of English Usage*, 1989).

decrease in metabolism with its attendant reduction in oxygen consumption is an effective response in these cases.

In hypothermia below 35°C, all physiological activity decreases: the pulse, blood pressure, and metabolism. In surgery, this is useful, since it reduces the need for oxygen by 40% (Cecil & Loeb, 1972). We observe that the somatic changes registered as effective in hibernation are similar to the somatic manifestations in depression or in its minor forms, dispiritedness and discouragement.[11]

As we know, the affect is equivalent to a universal and congenital hysterical attack (Freud, 1926d); it is the repetition of a motor activity that was formerly appropriate but is no longer. We can therefore assume that those somatic manifestations of depression are an inexpedient reaction—in the sense we have used when we discussed the theory of the affects—as the product of an unconscious confusion between spiritual privation and the privation of nutritive elements.

C. DISCOURAGEMENT AS A REACTION LACKING EXPEDIENCY IN THE PRESENT

As indicated above, the frustration of the need for spiritual exchange, attributed to a hostile environment, an adverse atmosphere, can generate the particular affect that we call discouragement as a process of discharge lacking expediency in the present. The person who is discouraged feels powerless to satisfy his own aspirations for love, attention, care, or appreciation, a deficit felt as if it were a lack of air, a situation that corresponds to the expression, "It [i.e., a snub] knocked the wind out of my sails." The person then resorts, automatically and unconsciously, to the reaction of discouragement as a form of dispiritedness, which was phylogenetically appropriate when the object of need at that particular stage—air—was lacking, yet inexpedient in the present when the nature of the need has changed: it is no longer air but, for example, a compliment.

As we have said, "to be encouraged" is to have the disposition and the inspiration for undertaking something, which requires among other things having a representation of the actions that must be taken in order to do it. This anticipatory image of the actions that must be done is what we could call a "proto-action," which is not to be confused with an ideal, an illusion, an "aspiration," or a "wish."

When a person feels she possesses the appropriate schemes of actions or is hopeful that her schemes of action will be effective, she feels

---

[11]"Listlessness" is also related to "dispiritedness." "Listless" derives from "lust," which in old Anglo-Saxon meant "pleasure." Obstfeld et al. (1982) suggest that "listlessness" refers to lack of desire to incorporate external objects, i.e., is related to receiving; dispiritedness, as a lack of spirits—the principle of human activity—is related to giving. The description of the state to which medicine gives the unusual name "asthenobiosis" is striking: reduced biological activity as in hibernation which neither depends on nor is related to temperature or humidity (*Dorland's Diccionario de Ciencias Médicas*, 1985).

encouraged. In this sense, we consider that breath, which corresponds to pulmonary respiration, is assigned the representation of the pleasurable affective state experienced when action schemes (proto-actions) function properly. On the other hand, as we have said, breath is also assigned the representation of the spirit for doing the action. For this reason, discouragement not only arises when patterns for action fail or because the action is more difficult than what had been supposed, but also because the search for new patterns is "discouraged." We tend to consider discouragement an affective state with negative connotations, but sometimes the action of discouraging has a positive aspect. In certain circumstances, "to discourage" a potentially harmful desire or behavior acquires the meaning of a protective attitude.

D. The Destructuring of the Affect "Discouragement"

What we know as "discouragement" and experience as a lack of willingness for action often becomes conscious without knowledge of the unconscious reasons. We believe that sometimes repression dislodges from consciousness not only the reasons for the discouragement but also the discouragement itself. In this case (experience has shown that this also happens with other affects), a recourse for avoiding the feeling of discouragement, which is unbearable to the conscious mind, consists in deforming its innervation key so that one of the elements of that key attracts upon itself the entire cathexis and it alone reaches consciousness, deprived of the original affective meaning.

As we have said, the elements with priority for receiving that cathexis are those that form the respiratory function. Thus, what comes to consciousness as a respiratory disorder may be considered an expression of the affect of discouragement: as the affect is not able to reach consciousness as such, its innervation key is destructured.

The disorder of the pulmonary respiratory function called dyspnea can be interpreted as a development equivalent to the affect of discouragement, a disorder that results from the pathosomatic deformation of the corresponding innervation key. The disorder is defined as dyspnea when consciousness categorizes it as a somatic process—deprived of affective meaning—or as a particular form of discouragement when consciousness interprets it as a psychical event.

E. Different Forms of "Discouragement"

According to our thesis, normal respiratory function is accompanied by the experience of "being encouraged." Therefore, "being encouraged" is accompanied by normal respiratory function, which is unconscious and therefore unnamed. When being discouraged reaches consciousness, it acquires the category of a feeling that can be recognized as such in its different aspects. The different respiratory disorders, on the other hand, represent, we believe, different forms of unconscious discouragement.

Discouragement can be expressed symbolically in two ways in the respiratory disorders in which difficulties related to inspiration predominate. The first is the feeling of being neglected or excluded from a social environment, which is generally symbolized by reference to the lack of "air" that has been "removed"; the above-cited expression, "It knocked the wind out of my sails," exemplifies this. The second mode corresponds to the feeling of not receiving the support or stimulus necessary for undertaking an action. This is evident in the expression, "They haven't encouraged me to do that."[12]

There is a form of discouragement that places emphasis on the expiratory phase. It forms the feeling of drowning, suffocation, or strangling that is experienced in a close relationship with symbiotic characteristics that thwarts vital and creative activities, a relationship that we call "asphyxiating." Another form of discouragement, which places the accent on respiratory rhythm, can be expressed or symbolized by heavy dyspneic respiration. In Spanish, *anhelar*, "to yearn," means "to breathe with difficulty" (meaning dyspnea) and also "to have a vehement wish or desire to get something" (Real Academia Española, 1950). Here too, the coexistence of both meanings in one word leads us to one common unconscious nucleus. If we accept that yearning implies hope and that hope corresponds to the defensive idealization of waiting[13] (Chiozza, 1963) by an individual who has lost confidence in the realization of what is desired (despair), then we find another reason for asserting that yearning conceals discouragement (Chiozza, 1981).

VII. SUMMARY OF THE SPECIFIC FANTASY
OF RESPIRATION

1. Like any other physiological function, what we consciously call metabolic and pulmonary respiration acquires its form from a specific unconscious structural matrix.

2. In the case of metabolic respiration, what reaches the conscious mind from the common unconscious matrix is, on the one hand, the

---

[12]This expression in Spanish is linked to respiration through the word *aliento*, which means "breath" and "encouragement." Analogously, we use the same word, *desaliento*, for "lack of breath" and for "discouragement." When we use the word "discouragement" in this chapter, the reader is asked to bear in mind both meanings of *desaliento*.

[13]In Spanish we use the word *esperar* both for "to wait" and "to hope." *Desesperar* is the term for despair (one stops hoping/waiting). Although these meanings are not linked in other languages, each language does have a word to refer to one of the aspects of the object/concept described. Accordingly, we hold that regardless of a person's language, in the unconscious, the meanings "wait," "hope," and "despair" are linked, so that reference to one of the aspects of this concept activates the others as well in the unconscious.

perception of the energy derived from metabolic processes and on the other, that disposition to action that we call *spirits*. For that reason, metabolic respiration can be assigned the representation of spirit and of the corresponding affective state we call "being in good spirits."

3. In the case of pulmonary respiration, what reaches the conscious system from a common unconscious matrix is, on the one hand, the feelings and perceptions corresponding to breath as a product of pulmonary respiration and on the other, that particular experience of receiving encouragement implicit in the meaning of the Spanish verb *alentar*, "to encourage." For this reason, pulmonary respiration can be assigned the representation of "breath" and the corresponding affective state, to the meaning of the word "encouraged."

4. While being encouraged and spirited are unconscious, discouragement and dispiritedness are typical and universal affects which frequently reach the conscious mind and are experienced consciously as feelings. These feelings are named "discouragement" and "dispiritedness," precisely because the disorders that lead to what the conscious mind categorizes as lack of air or energy are assigned the representation of the complete affective process, since the unconscious structural matrix of the pulmonary and metabolic respiratory function is part of the innervation key of that affective process.

5. Pulmonary inspiration is assigned the representation of the inspiration that encourages creation and becomes a symbol of that part of the creative act. This is evident in the use of the same word to represent both processes and in the fact that, both in myths and in literature, the act of creation is represented by the participation of air, wind, or an "encouraging" breeze which animates matter. We also find the word "aspiration" in language linked to the inspiration of respiratory physiology. It is assigned the representation of desire, yearning, or the impulse to achieve something, as shown in the use of the same word to represent both processes.

Pulmonary respiration mainly designates the entry of air into the lungs; aspiration, on the other hand, as a physiological process, mainly designates the act by which air is removed from a given place. Creative inspiration accompanies the act of creating a work; aspiration as an experience, on the other, accompanies a desire that has not been realized.

6. Inspired air, "breath," or "pneuma" symbolizes the soul and the spirit, as many examples taken from etymology and mythology demonstrate. Therefore, normal pulmonary respiratory functioning, which implies exchange of gases with the environment, is assigned the representation of good social and spiritual exchange with the objects in the environment. For this very reason, the same word, *atmosphere*, is used to refer to shared space, both physical and social.

The expression "to breeze through" has the meaning of emerging successfully from a situation involving struggle, embarrassment, offense, or a rebuff. Breathing fully symbolizes, in that linguistic form, feeling spiritually satisfied at having overcome a difficulty.

7. The affect of discouragement can be expressed symbolically in two different ways. One of these, predominantly inspiratory, can take either of two forms. The first is the feeling of being neglected or excluded from the social environment, symbolized by air that is absent because it has been taken away, as shown in the choice of the word "rebuff" (in Spanish, literally "dis-air") to refer to this type of rejection or disdain. The second corresponds to the feeling of not receiving the support or stimulus necessary for undertaking an action, symbolized by air that is lacking because it has not been granted, as in the expression, "They haven't encouraged me to do that."

The other, predominantly expiratory, forms the feeling of drowning, suffocation, or strangulation that is experienced in a close relationship with symbiotic characteristics that thwarts the realization of vital activities and creativity, linked to what we customarily call "asphyxiation."

8. The sigh, preceded by a situation in which "breath has been thwarted," is a heavy and prolonged inspiration followed by a prolonged expiration which is its special and audible representation. It is "respiration" that comes from deep within the soul, as reflected in the etymology of the word "sigh" in Spanish. If we take note that it comes after a moment in which breathing is suspended, we can assume that it represents a "venting of one's feelings" that expresses the overcoming of discouragement.

9. Biology interprets hibernation, characterized by decrease in metabolism and temperature and by minimum oxygen consumption, as an archaic response to the external lack of nutrients in the environment, indispensable for vital functions. Hibernation provides the phylogenetic model that forms the innervation key of the affect of discouragement.

When frustration of the demand for social and spiritual exchange is, in the conscious mind, erroneously and symbolically interpreted as lack of food and oxygen, the affect of discouragement arises as a phylogenetically appropriate motor act (hibernation) which is, however, ineffective in the present. It also represents, symbolically, an attempt to bring to the present the prenatal stage, preserving the omnipotent fantasy of not being dependent on exchange with the external environment. The discouragement of an action or a desire can, however, obviously function as a form of projection in certain circumstances.

10. Dyspnea can be interpreted as a development equivalent to the affect of discouragement, which results from the pathosomatic deformation of its innervation key. The disorder is experienced as dyspnea when the conscious system categorizes it as a somatic process—lacking affective meaning—or as a particular form of discouragement when the conscious system interprets it as a psychical event.

11. The verb *anhelar*, "to yearn," means: to have the vehement desire to attain something and also, in Spanish, to breathe with difficulty. For this reason, "yearning" respiration, a particular form of dyspnea, is assigned the representation of a vehement desire which is usually constituted as a reaction formation to discouragement.

VIII. The Meanings of Asthma

A. Review of the Literature

T. French and F. Alexander (quoted by Canteros in Abadi [1968]) maintain that since respiration is the first postnatal function, it represents the child's biological independence from the mother. Thus, the dyspneic crisis expresses both the need for protection and a protest against the relation of excessive dependency. The determinants of the attack are associated with situations of fear and anger, with situations that threaten the relation of dependency and the security based on it, and with sexual conflicts. The feared separation from the mother, which threatens dependency and security, is not a real physical separation but the danger of losing closeness with the mother because of a temptation to which the patient is exposed; the asthma attack seems to mean a suppressed scream and a suffocated confession addressed to the mother. The authors emphasize that the precipitating situation is formed by indecision and conflict between adhering to and separating from the mother. The reasons for the inhibition of the scream are attributed to the maternal demand for premature independent and self-sufficient attitudes, as well as the tendency opposed to excessive maternal dependency. The asthma attack also expresses a protest against separation and the need to get oxygen independently, as well as a protest against the desire to reestablish dependency on the mother by crying (or screaming). The mother of the asthmatic has been characterized as narcissistic, ambitious, and not very maternal. The parents are described as passive and detached from their children and the asthmatic child as being uniformly stubborn, exhibitionistic, and demanding.

Weizsaecker found vengeful stubbornness to be a character trait of asthmatic patients. He stated that such stubbornness arises from the fear of losing security: "The asthmatic attack is a kind of scene of weeping that takes place in the lungs, as an expression of fear, stubbornness and of that threat of illness and death" (1950a, p. 86). Referring to what one psychologist said about a patient, he described how her "mother-imago" received a hard blow that damaged her spirits. He added that in asthma the patient cries and shouts from the deepest level of the lungs and concluded by remarking that "The physiological functions in asthma reflect something of the passionate forces that are more effective in the spirit than the logical and intellectual ones."

H. Racker (1948) argued that birth marks the moment of the first frustration, since it breaks the identity between subject and object; from then on, the object and the bad remain equivalents. Analyzing several asthmatic patients, he found that they inhibited loving, because they experienced it as a loss of libido from the ego, equivalent to death. These patients feel in danger of being absorbed (loved, eaten, killed) by the Molok-mother[14] and have to defend themselves from it.

Thus, the following appears:

1. A conflict between incorporating (loving, eating, having inside, being united, being saved from death) the mother and not incorporating her (avoiding the bad, death, and also dying from lack of her breast).
2. A struggle between the patient and the mother, who wants to get in through his/her respiratory system. The defense consists in closing the bronchi.
3. Another defense consists in incorporating the object and setting up a conflict between retaining the mother and ejecting her.
4. Out of fear of being absorbed, the attempt (with death anxiety) to be filled again and also to eliminate the dangerous object. The asthmatic tries to achieve both by inspiring the object. Since it is a bad object, it must be attacked. The asthma attack therefore becomes a "melancholic process" in the respiratory apparatus, as described by Pichon-Rivière (1943).
5. The patient has introjected the object which attacks and kills him/her from within. In this sense, asthma is a somatic conversion in a delusion of suffocating. The fact that the object is "inspired" represents the attempt to incorporate it, avoiding oral aggressiveness. The sneeze is a rejection of the object by the nose, which elicits a "Bless you" and is felt as a form of external support.

For asthmatics, the mother is equivalent to air. Both inspiration and expiration are deadly, and the patient "suffocates, dies" in this conflict. Suffocating is equivalent to lack of air and to having lost the mother. The contradiction between independence and passivity can be understood on a deeper level: that of birth. Being born is separating from the mother and dying. But being born is also living. Not being born is also death, but it is being united to the mother and therefore living. This is what the asthmatic finally chooses.

O. Fenichel (1957) referred to bronchial asthma as an organ neurosis of the respiratory apparatus. In bronchial asthma, it is especially a (passive-receptive) yearning for the mother that the pathological alterations

---

[14]Racker used the idea of the Molok-mother to refer to the image of an "absorbing mother" who gives and at the same time sucks. Molok was a Phoenician god who, like Saturn, ate children.

of the respiratory function express. The asthma attack is above all an equivalent to anxiety, which is perceived as a fear of asphyxia, a scream for help addressed to the mother whom the patient tries to introject by respiration in order to be permanently protected. The anal orientation of the patients in general has developed from an interest in smelling into an interest in breathing.

Arminda Aberastury (1951) observed that asthmatic children construct houses with a great many small windows located high up, symbolizing the difficulty in breathing. Adriana, a girl who began to have asthma attacks at the age of eight when her brother was born, displacing her from her place as "the youngest," represented the feeling of suffocating by drawing a figure in which the arms grew out of the throat. Other children who suffered severe attacks would break part of a wall of the house they constructed, leaving a hole through which air could enter.

A line of investigation begun by M. Abadi (1968) and followed by Cagnoni (1971) links respiration with birth. Abadi discussed the image of a sphinx mother who retains the child and does not allow it to be born, thus threatening it with suffocation. He described the absence of a good father who, taking the role of a midwife, will help the child to be born and rescue it from its confinement within the mother. According to these ideas, he regarded the asthma attack as a repetition of the traumatic situation of the impeded birth. According to this author, the asthmatic feels confined and suffocated by its sphinx-mother. According to Cagnoni, "breathing is having a soul because it is being born and this is equivalent to coming out of death, to which the mother who impedes birth has condemned the child" (Cagnoni, 1971, p. 4).

Using the method of investigating the specific fantasies, N. Canteros (1979) hypothesized that in asthma there are exudative, allergic, and spasmodic fantasies and that this combination of fantasies, which we refer to as a "mosaic," also includes a pulmonary fantasy. The author maintains that

> In his crisis of expiratory dyspnea, the asthmatic is stubbornly refusing to carry out a multiple exchange that frightens him and tries, by means of the retained air, secretions and exudates, to realize the wish to preserve the symbiotic relationship as if it were a prenatal situation. What he tries to avoid in this realization of desire is the feeling of fright, loneliness and responsibility that accompanies the process of birth-individuation. [1979, p. 24]

She emphasized the link between the attack of dyspnea and catastrophic anxiety. She pointed out that this feeling does not come into the asthmatic's consciousness and that dyspnea arises instead. She asserted that in the asthma attack, patients repeat a pattern based on the act of birth. Thus, there are two stages in the attack: the first one is retentive symbiotic, and is analogous to what happens when labor is obstructed or indolent, and the second stage, like the act of birth itself, is an abrupt tearing away, which leads the patient to experience extreme hopelessness and to develop catastrophic anxiety. She considered the bronchial narrowing and the retention of air as the expression of the realization of a desire: that of recreating the first stage of the act of birth, that is, of retentive prenatal symbiosis. If his attack enables the asthmatic to experience the fantasy of still being in the womb, he/she avoids feeling the traumatic anxiety that birth involves.

According to our investigations (Chiozza et al., 1987), all pulmonary respiratory disorders are the expression of the "discouragement" affect, which, failing to reach consciousness, has been deformed in its innervation key. The affect can be expressed symbolically in two different ways—one in which the inspiratory phase of respiration predominates and the other, in which exhalation predominates. The latter comprises the feelings of choking, suffocating, or strangling that are experienced in a close relationship with symbiotic characteristics, which impedes the carrying out of vital activities and creativity, as in the kind of relationship we usually call "asphyxiating." Asthma is the main illness among those who express the fantasies corresponding to exhalation-predominant discouragement.

B. ASTHMATIC DYSPNEA

The clinical picture of bronchial asthma is characterized by bronchial spasm leading to expiratory dyspnea and by the presence of an alveolar exudate. The alveolar exudate can be understood as the pathosomatic[15] expression of vicarious weeping. Asthmatic dyspnea, on the other hand, presupposes the establishment of the following conditions:

1. A current frustration at the attained level of death-libido development[16] and regression to a neonatal respiratory point of fixation.[17]

---

[15]Together with neurosis and psychosis as psychical disorders, we include "pathosomatosis," which manifests itself as a corporeal disorder. Pathosomatic repression of an affect is accomplished by a displacement of cathexis that occurs inside the innervation key.

[16]With respect to "death-libido development," in *Psychoanalysis of the Hepatic Disorders*, Chiozza (1963) stated that along with libidinal development, Freud pointed to an evolution in the expression of death instinct. This allows us to speak of death-libido development insofar as the different forms of primacy of the stages of the libido determine different ways in which instinctual fusion takes place.

[17]With regard to the "neonatal respiratory point of fixation," Freud remarked upon the fixation of an instinct at some particular point in its development and also stated that every important process can become an erogenous zone. He also maintained that the primacy of an erogenous zone was established during libidinal development, for example, oral primacy, thus allowing for a "point of fixation." Chiozza, in *Psychoanalysis of the Hepatic Disorders* (1963), on the basis of these Freudian concepts, stated that it is possible to find primacies and points of fixation other than those classically described.

At this level, normal pulmonary respiratory function implies adequate exchange of gases (air) with the environment and good social and spiritual exchange with surrounding objects ("atmosphere"), which can be presented reciprocally through breath/encouragement used as a symbol. When there is a respiratory regression, the current frustration of an affective demand is experienced as pressing, like the need for oxygen, and the relationship with the object acquires characteristics similar to those of symbiosis. The lack of a good social context is then experienced as the absence of an encouraging and yearned-for object, always considered equivalent to the presence of a hostile environment that "discourages."

2. A "symbiotic" relationship with an object that the person experiences as a continuous threat of being deserted, while at the same time it must satisfy a peremptory need.

On the respiratory level, this desertion is experienced as the "snub" of a discouraging object and the expiratory phase of normal respiration can be confused, in the unconscious, with a way of running the risk of desertion.

3. An attempt to retain that object of yearning, an attempt that, in the subject's experience, increases its frustrating nature, since its retention does not diminish the "discouragement."

Just as the retained air loses its oxygen content and impedes obtaining new, oxygenated air, the object retained at a level of respiratory regression is experienced as a bad object that blocks the functioning of vital activities and the subject's creativity. Because of the respiratory regression, such an object-relationship evokes the expiratory type of the affect of discouragement: the absence of an encouraging object is made equivalent in the unconscious to the presence of an object that chokes, asphyxiates, or strangles.

4. The impossibility of the affect of discouragement reaching consciousness.
5. The destructuring of the innervation key of discouragement and its symbolic representation by one of the elements of that innervation key: dyspnea, which attracts the total intensity of the cathexis upon itself and reaches consciousness as a somatic phenomenon deprived of its affective meaning.

Thus, it becomes a development equivalent to the affect of discouragement.

IX. Case Material

A. Monica (22 years old)

Monica, a student of architecture, consulted us because of an asthma attack that required hospitalization and use of an oxygen mask. The affection she feels for Gus, her boyfriend, is not the love she felt for John, with whom she had her first sexual intercourse at age 15. They often fight, because he is a dreamer and his feet aren't on the ground. Gus has now suggested that they live together to try it out. Monica does not feel protected, because she feels he is as unstable and weak like a child.

Monica's family approves of their living together and has even offered her an apartment, but she doesn't know what to do. She feels that her family is unaware of her insecurity, fears, and doubts. She experiences their attitude as a desertion and would like them to understand her and help her to decide; she feels increasingly anxious.

Since she was a child, she has felt the desire for someone to always be at her side, unconditionally. She had her first asthma attack when she was three, when her parents separated. Monica was sleeping with her mother at that time, but even so, she felt her mother was far away. Her mother . . . was always busy with her profession and didn't like to keep house. She felt constantly threatened by the feeling that her mother would desert her. Her father was no secure presence either. He remarried and Monica's bed was given away to Adriana, Daddy's wife's daughter. Monica grew up strongly attached to her mother and still clings to the illusion of having her there forever, but when she tells her about her things and Mummy gives her opinion, Monica begins to feel that she intrudes too much in her life, that she has to stop her. It is her mother who gives her her apartment, tells her what she should do, and without asking permission lends her bedroom to the relatives who come to visit them.

On the day of the latest attack, they were celebrating Christmas all together. There was a strange atmosphere, an asphyxiating atmosphere. Her cousins, haughty and deprecating, came to visit and used "her" things and "her" home. One of the smaller cousins played with her guitar and broke it. She felt increasingly anxious, nervous, impotent, invaded, and misunderstood. Her mother and Paul, her husband, left the room after lunch to have a nap. Gus also went to sleep, leaving her alone. She then remembered that her godmother was in the hospital because of a crisis of depression and was afraid of ending up like her. Suddenly, she felt that she couldn't breathe, that she was choking. That was the beginning of the asthma attack that led to the consultation.

The contrast that she establishes between the scene of her mother and Paul enjoying their nap in the same bed on the day of the attack and her "desertion" by Gus, who sleeps alone, appropriately dramatizes Monica's disappointment about the imminent "marriage," which does not enthuse her. This current frustration and the respiratory regression that it triggers in Monica fulfill the first condition for the emergence of her "somatic" illness.

Monica's respiratory regression can be seen not only in the fact that she experiences her family environment as an asphyxiating atmosphere but also, especially, in the peremptory nature of her feeling of needing the objects with which she establishes a quasi-symbiotic relationship. She needs them "as air" and experiences frustration on this level and the feeling of being snubbed, which "discourages" her.

The second condition for the establishment of a respiratory dyspnea, that the people taken as objects of a peremptory need are at the same time experienced as objects that constantly threaten to desert her, can be seen clearly in Monica's history. She feels that her mother, the only "close" person since her parents' separation, is "far away." This type of relationship, characterized by a yearning to "breeze through" that culminates in the snub, is symbolized in the fact that they suddenly take her bed away, and this is repeated in her most intimate and meaningful relationships, for example, in her dependency on Gus, who "discourages" her and fails to "inspire" her enthusiasm.

Monica not only preserves the illusion of having mother with her forever but also attempts to retain her so that she doesn't desert her. For that reason, she tells her about her life, although for some time now she has "known" that she cannot understand. Therefore, she feels that her "retained" mother invades her, "prying into her life" without understanding, deciding upon her life in a way that makes her feel "asphyxiated." Here we see the third condition for the development of an expiratory dyspnea. The patient attempts to defend herself from discouragement and dispiritedness but is incapable of "letting go" of the object; instead of "breezing through," she "chokes."

The fear of anger, of fighting, of the risk of being deserted, but above all, the deep-rooted conviction of being extremely helpless that is incompatible with life, a conviction that is only obscurely revealed at times in Monica's anguish over the idea of solitude, must have combined so that her conscious mind could not bear the affective discouragement that she experiences in her most intimate relationships.

Monica's affective discouragement is evident in her consciousness as a dyspnea that she prefers to attribute to a "somatic" origin because, in this way, besides avoiding the traumatic feeling of bringing into consciousness the circumstances in which she felt the discouragement, she avoids the unbearable experience of discouragement itself.

The intensity of the regression, which determines the intensity of the affective experience, renders necessary the defensive deformation of the innervation key of the affect involved; at the same time, it facilitates that deformation by way of the very intensity of the cathexes. In other words, at this level of regression, in which the mother is like the air she breathes, she cannot make her lack conscious, but precisely for this reason, she represents her lacking/want as a lack of air.

B. HUGO (39 YEARS OLD)

The diagnosis was "chronic obstructive bronchopulmonary disease." He had emphysema. . . . He had had bronchial asthma since he was two, and the bronchitis contracted five years ago had never gone away. . . .

He always tried to seem optimistic, active, euphoric, but lately he had had too much unpleasantness. . . .

When his brothers came to Buenos Aires at the end of last year, everything should have been like it was before: the four together with Mom . . . but the reproaches started . . . and they ended up with a fight that left a bitter taste in his mouth. . . . The image of the united family vanished. . . . The New Year's party that he had always given in his house was perhaps no longer worth it. . . .

He wanted to have more children. . . . Over the summer vacation, he had suggested that Ronny take out her diaphragm forever. . . . She, perhaps more realistic, had told him that it wasn't a good idea until he was better . . . that when the twins were born he had started his bronchitis and that she had had to take care of the twins and of him too.

His friend and sidekick, Peter, his university classmate and partner since they had graduated as engineers, now develops his own projects. . . .

Ronny isn't the same anymore either. . . . She's very busy . . . with the children who started school, and the institute . . . that she's just opened. . . . At night she gets home exhausted . . . doesn't feel like starting love play. . . . In bed, he feels tremendously cold all over, and every time he coughs he has to spit. . . . He musn't forget to take his handkerchief with him! . . . and the bronchodilator . . . just in case. . . .

He kisses her less too. . . . He doesn't laugh like he used to . . . but it's for fear of getting out of breath . . . (and of his bad breath!). . . . He coughs more and more. . . . He gets more and more out of breath . . . he's weaker and weaker . . . and thinner too!

His childhood, in spite of the asthma, had been a happy time. Mom was the one who was always there . . . the spirit of the home . . . paying attention to any change in his childhood illness. . . . She was the one who understood him . . . although, almost always, she imposed her tastes on him and he wasn't able to react. . . . When he had just graduated, he married Ronny, they went to live in the States. Those were good times. . . . The bronchitis started when they returned. . . . They wanted the twins to be born here.

Mom wasn't the same anymore . . . he found her more distant, into her own things. . . . She didn't behave like the grandmother he had hoped to offer his children . . . a grandmother like the one he had had. . . . His friends had also changed a lot . . . interested in their own lives . . . they weren't the ones he had dreamt of coming back to. . . . Then, at the moment when, lonelier than he had ever been, he was going to be a father, he felt, in his flesh, the hole that his father's death left in his life. From lung cancer . . . when Hugo was twenty-six.

Dad had never been strong; when he was still a boy, it was Mom who had taught him things about sex and birth . . . so that he would know about it! . . . without thinking about the consequences . . . without calculating the emotions he might feel. . . .

He still remembers the eyes all around him that looked at him in the dark of his room when, full of anguish, he stayed in bed not daring to call out . . . and he also remembers that in adolescence he decided to leave his first girlfriend because Mom didn't like her.

There's no point in repeating over and over again that "he walks above earthly reality." There's no point in denying that when he gets home and has to eat alone, he watches any old thing on TV. . . .

He feels very thin and very weak . . . nearly prostrated . . . but Ronny's there . . . she's a tractor . . . she's got a capacity for hard work that's marvelous . . . incredible vigor . . . the initiative is all hers.

Ronny is more and more enthused with her new occupations and no longer wants to start love play. He also kisses her less and laughs less, to avoid the wheezing and for fear of the bad breath. Thus, Hugo tells us of his current genital frustration, which necessitates his regression to the points of fixation at which most of his libido had been arrested during development.

Apparently, the feeling of weakness that has always pursued him, now displaced onto his extreme thinness, symbolized by the hole that the death of his father left in him, led him to adopt an infantile position in relation to his wife. However, an intense fixation to neonatal respiratory primacy enables us to better understand the vicissitudes of the relationships that Hugo has established. His need for the object is as peremptory as that for the air he breathes. The threat of desertion contained in Ronny's genital listlessness, which Hugo also reads in the fact that she does not want to have more children, is experienced on this respiratory level as a snub that produces discouragement.

Something similar happens when he returned from the States and found his mother more distant, "into her own things" and his friends very much changed, each "into his own thing."

The attempt to retain that object of a peremptory yearning, an object that snubs at the same time, does not diminish the discouragement; to the contrary, it is experienced as the presence of a bad object that invades, chokes, and asphyxiates; an object impossible to exhale.

Hugo suffers "somatically" because of the old and retained air in the expiratory dyspnea, the emphysema, and the obstructive bronchitis, whose exudates symbolize repressed weeping vicariously expressed.

He prefers to interpret his suffering as a "somatic symptom" because he needs to keep unconscious the particular type of ill-being that he feels when Ronny, like his mother, imposes her will, her desires, her way of life, her schedules.

If the experience of submission were to reach his consciousness, he would be forced to face the fear of desertion and the extreme dependency that keeps him from reacting; but facing this is nearly impossible for him, since in his unconscious, desertion is confused with a terrifying experience of asphyxiation; what returns of it in each episode of asthmatic dyspnea is only a small "sample."

C. MARION (30 YEARS OF AGE)

When she met John five years ago, she felt trapped. With Robert, the manager of the company where she worked, she had had sexual intercourse for the first time . . . she needed him very much. . . . the idea of doing it with another man inspired a feeling of violence in her . . . but with him there was no future. . . . Robert had no intention of separating from his family . . . he would never be totally hers. . . . she could neither go on nor break off. . . .

She had seen that John was . . . quite alone . . . and had wanted to help him . . . she could be his lifesaver! When John suggested that they take a trip together, she stopped seeing Robert . . . although she never stopped loving him. . . .

Though with John things weren't perfect—their sex life wasn't good—she had found someone who could be "hers," who saw her as a "good girl," serious, professional. . . . She felt she was on top of the world. . . . Perhaps a certain concession in sex was part of what she had to give up in order to be a bride. . . .

It's true that sometimes he was a bit contradictory, he suggested and decided, but you never knew what he was going to do in the end . . . maybe with time, she would eventually feel more sure of being someone important for him. . . . She had to become important for him (!) . . . because the idea of solitude seemed simply unbearable to her.

At that time, on top of it all, she started to be ill . . . before the abortion, the bronchitis, and then the first of her asthma attacks. . . . It was impossible to go on with the pregnancy! . . . They hardly knew each other at that time. Shortly after the abortion, they married, not realizing that she was pregnant again. . . . When Frederick was born, John got fired . . . and the fights over things that were hard to remember began. . . . God only knows that she fought to keep her illusions, the same ones she had at the beginning, when although he was authoritarian and she submitted, everything was idyllic.

In spite of the fights, they were together then, but the distance was enormous. . . . She felt lonely, tortured by painful humiliation . . . and by dry-eyed weeping, like that time in the train station, when she was fourteen and her boyfriend returned from his school trip and got off the train with the girl who had taken her place.

How awful she had felt! . . . hesitating between awkwardness, the feeling of being an ugly duckling, and the injustice . . . that had pursued her since she was a child . . . in spite of the perfect homework that her mother demanded of her in an authoritarian manner, her mother who seemed to be faultless. . . . How awful she had felt in the nuns' school . . . where thinking about being a woman was a sin. . . .

And yet, though she felt insignificant in the eyes of her "sexier" girlfriends, who didn't dress like little girls, Ralph, the boy they all wanted, had come to her to be his girlfriend . . . before dropping her there on the platform . . . the same year that, without saying good-bye, her father died of lung cancer . . . just when she was beginning to become his sidekick. . . .

She had gone away, with John, for a few days to Mendoza, in a useless attempt to re-create a good atmosphere. When they came back, she got pneumonia. . . .

And after the pneumonia she went back to work . . . but it was hard to relate to people. She had lost the joy and the initiative she had had when she was an adolescent, when she was the leader of her schoolmates in school and at university . . . she had always wanted to do something transcendent. . . .

Alone . . . in the big house they built with so many illusions . . . with a beautiful garden . . . and a newborn baby . . . but in the suburbs, with no car and no phone, now that she no longer works and feels confined, it's hard to bear John's being at work in the city all day long . . . his acting indifferently . . . and getting back later and later! . . .

Besides, the pneumonia came back and the asthma has worsened. . . . She tried again, as she had been doing since she was small . . . and again she was in the same dead-end situation, where she is trapped. . . .

Marion, submissive in her relationship with Robert, which she felt was a constant snub from an object that she couldn't retain, that wasn't hers, could only do without him because she managed to breeze through, replacing him with John, since the idea of solitude seemed simply unbearable to her.

John, whom she had thought to be very lonely, would never desert her because he, as if about to choke, would need her; however, John, who could be "retained," rapidly became bad: she thinks that perhaps with time she would feel more sure of being someone important for him and adds that she had to do it. At the same time the fights over things that were difficult to remember began.

In this part of her history, we see the second and third conditions for the existence of an expiratory dyspnea: her experience that the object of a peremptory need threatens her again with desertion and the failed attempt to diminish the discouragement by retaining that object, which thus becomes a suffocating presence.

Meanwhile, Robert again became the yearned-for object, now becoming the man whom she never stopped loving, since with John sex wasn't good but a certain concession in sex in order to be a bride had been necessary.

In this way, Marion clearly expresses that she gives up part of her genitality in order to decrease the danger of being deserted; but the genital frustration, which increases the regression and constitutes the first condition in this case for the establishment of the bronchial asthma, increases the fear of desertion and the suffering from an asphyxiating relationship.

Her asthma attacks at this time correspond to the fact that the intensity of the affects involved leads to the repression of discouragement, thus transforming it by deforming its innervation key into an expiratory dyspnea.

Marion's two episodes of pneumonia show us, on the other hand, the operation of different fantasies. She was looking for a beautiful garden, a symbol of air, that represents, on a level of respiratory regression, a good exchange with persons in the environment who, for her, are objects of a peremptory need. Her attempt to re-create a good atmosphere to recover the atmosphere of adolescent joy that she had lost was defeated by repetition compulsion. Tortured by "dry-eyed weeping" and angry with John, who returns later and later, she suddenly found that the emotional distance was enormous. She was alone, confined, with no car and no phone, no communication, feeling that it was difficult to relate to people, farther and farther from something transcendent for her.

4

THE SPECIFIC UNCONSCIOUS MEANINGS OF VARICOSE VEINS

L. A. CHIOZZA, G. L. DE BALDINO,
LILIANA C. DE GRUS, H. SCHUPACK

I. INTRODUCTION

Varicose veins (from the Greek *uarix*, "dilation," "dilated vein") are abnormally dilated and twisted peripheral veins (Foote, 1969; Del Campo Llerena, 1984), which sometimes appear in the skin, where they are visible to the naked eye.

Del Campo Llerena (1984) asserted that varicose veins respond to pathophysiological factors that are similar throughout the body, although he devoted chapters to pathology, as in varicose veins of the esophagus, varicocele, hemorrhoids, and the like. The *primum movens* of superficial or peripheral venous insufficiency is hyperdistensibility of the vein wall, which provokes valvular incontinence; this in turn worsens the dilation of the wall. The consequences are reflux, venous stasis, and the formation of varicose veins.

Just as medicine describes factors that are common to the different types of varicose veins, from the point of view of the psychoanalytic approach to somatic illness, we find specific unconscious meanings that characterize the varicose disorder and differentiate it from other pathological conditions. We shall try to understand varicose veins as the physical aspect of specific fantasies, to develop some ideas linked to the specific meanings of this illness, and to broach the understanding of one of its particular forms, varicose veins of the lower limbs.

II. Varicose Veins from the Medical Viewpoint

A. The Venous System

The most important function of the veins is to enable blood to return from the tissues and flow toward the heart; the portal systems are an exception, since they convey venous blood first to other organs (e.g., the liver). Normally, the direction of the circulation is from the periphery toward the heart, and from the superficial vascular toward the deep vascular network. The venous valves serve to prevent venous reflux (Del Campo Llerena, 1984).

Other functions are to participate in temperature regulation (i.e., dermal, subdermal, and subcutaneous veins with sympathetic innervation) and to serve as a reservoir for blood. The venous system contains between 70% and 80% of the total blood volume, which is mobilized as needed. Thus, sufficient filling of the cardiac chambers is assured in the intervals between contractions, and cardiac filling is, in its turn, a principal determinant of the volume of blood ejected by each ventricular contraction. For all these reasons, the venous system can be considered the dynamic modulator[1] of cardiac performance (Shephard & Vanhoutte, 1978).

B. Varicose Veins in the Lower Limbs

According to Pietravallo (1985), the tendency today is to use the concept of "phlebopathies" to designate venous disorders of the lower limbs, among which varicose veins (dilation of one or more tracts of the superficial system) are included. The term "phlebopathies" designates a general category of disorders of the venous system.

In the legs, the venous circulation comprises two systems: (1) superficial, which includes two main branches, the external and the internal saphenous vein, and (2) deep, formed by the deep veins: tibial, popliteal, femoral, etc., which follow the paths of the arteries with the same name. The two systems have widespread anastomoses in the foot and are partially independent in the leg and the thigh, where they are linked by piercing or communicating veins (Del Campo Llerena, 1984). Return flow of blood from the lower limbs is favored by: (a) the vis à tergo (i.e., the residue of arterial pressure), (b) the activity of the bellows of the chest muscles, (c) the venous valves, (d) the contraction of the muscular pump of the calf (the "peripheral venous heart"), and (e) evacuation during walking of the "venous

---

[1]This refers to the role of the dynamics of the venous system in the regulation of blood flow. The venous system contains 70–80% of the blood volume, and it assures adequate filling of the cardiac chambers during cardiac diastole. Acting as the "first factor" in determining cardiac output and pressure on the arterial side of the circulation, it can be viewed as the circulation's dynamic modulator.

sole" of Lejars (i.e., the venous "sponge" in the soles of the feet; cf. Pietravallo [1985]). Venous return is hindered by: (a) the force of gravity, (b) increased pressure in the abdomen and chest; and (c) the viscosity of the blood.

Varicose veins, or superficial phlebopathies of the lower limbs, can be congenital or acquired and are divided into two major groups: (1) primary, idiopathic, or essential, coexisting with normal function of the deep veins, and (2) secondary, a consequence of circulatory reflux into the superficial veins from the deep venous system through the communicating venous system. The common denominator in the latter group of disorders—post-thrombotic or postphlebitic varicose veins, those produced by abdominal-pelvic tumor compression, varicose veins secondary to arterial-venous fistulae, and the like—is venous hypertension.

Several factors are involved in the genesis of the phlebopathies: (a) predisposition, hereditary or congenital, to varicose veins, and (b) triggering or acquired factors. In the first category are heredity conditions such as the varicose diathesis, reflected in mesenchymatic weakness of the walls of the veins or in hypoplasia of the valves. This tendency is usually not limited to the veins, since several disorders may coexist: muscle hypotonia, dystrophy, flaccidity, hernia, flat feet, and so on (Lacour, 1981; Shephard & Vanhoutte, 1978). Some authors propose that the primary cause is the action of hormones of the estrogen group which, through the sympathetic system, produce hypotonia in the smooth muscles of the veins (Lacour, 1981). The most frequent triggering factors are those that produce repeated increments in abdominal pressure: prolonged standing position, sedentary life style, obesity, trauma, pregnancy, and so on.

The dystrophy of the walls and valves produces reflux from the region of the affected valve. The reflux acts progressively on the vein farthest from this region, producing a series of changes in its caliber (dilation and twisting) and its properties (loss of elasticity, resistance, fragility) (Barrow, 1948; Farreras Valenti & Rozman, 1982; Pietravallo, 1985). In turn, the weight of the column of liquid, poorly distributed because of the incompetent valves, increases dilation and stasis in unaffected sectors, generating a vicious circle (varicose progress) (Pietravallo, 1985). The stasis or vein reflux (stagnant blood that progressively loses O_2 and raises the CO_2 content) may explain the propensity to fatigue, pain, and cramps that patients report (Foote, 1969).

Varicose veins of the lower limbs are common. Around 10% of persons over 35 years of age suffer from varicose veins, the frequency being four times greater in women than in men. Patients usually seek medical help because of pain or swelling of the legs and for cosmetic improvement. In other cases, a complication of the varicose disorder—varicorrhagia, varicophlebitis, or trophic skin disorders—bring the patient to the physician. Neither the severity of the symptoms nor the magnitude of complications is proportional to the extent of varicose vein development since morphologically important varicose veins may be well tolerated and fail to cause major complications (Del Campo Llerena, 1984).

The treatment of varicose veins can include: (a) medication (anti-inflammatory agents and drugs to restore venous tone, to which the use of elastic bandages, the elevation of the feet during rest, massages, physical conditioning exercises, and the like can be added; (b) chemical agents that destroy the endothelial tissue of the varicose veins; and (c) surgery, with ligation of the insufficient vessels and resection of the varicose veins (Del Campo Llerena, 1984; Pietravallo, 1985).

III. VARICOSE VEINS AS ENCODING SPECIFIC FANTASIES

A. VENOUS RETURN

The heart is a vessel that has been differentiated to the point that it has become the central organ of the vascular system (Houssay, 1955). The great veins near the heart are subjected to rhythmic muscle contractions synchronously with cardiac activity.[2] Just as medicine proves the unity between veins and heart, the psychoanalytic view finds meanings that cardiac function shares with the venous system. The heart has from ancient times been considered "the seat of feelings," with its pacemaker, its beats, and its different rhythms and is therefore particularly apt for symbolizing the different emotional tones that give emotions their quality (Chiozza, 1978; Chiozza et al., 1982).

The heart also represents another mental factor: the process of remembering. Etymology shows the connections between linguistic forms pertaining to the heart and to memory: the Spanish word for "remember" (similar to the English "record") is composed of the prefix "re-," which denotes repetition, return, backward movement and of "cor/cordis," which means "heart" (Chiozza, 1978). The process of remembering—according to its customary denotation, which is equivalent to recall, memory, reminiscence, and the like—is a complex phenomenon that involves the presence of ideas, feelings, visual images, and affects. Various organs of the body could symbolize the different components of this process. Thus, for example, reminiscence (derived from "re": repeat, return, and from "mind") would involve the return of an idea to the mind, a mind that acquires its main corporeal representation in the brain. Taking into account the etymological sense of the Spanish word

---

[2]Some animals have veins whose periodic contractions are real beats. This is, for example, true of the veins of bats' wings (Houssay, 1955).

for "remember" and the English "record" would involve re-experiencing or re-feeling affects consciously referring to the past and implying a cardiac component.[3]

The vein-heart system (return circulation) is therefore specifically linked to the emotional aspect of memory.[4] Both the veins and the heart represent a complex process, of which they are an important part. In this sense, we could say in brief that we remember when the heart "re-feels" something that the vein (whose etymology is "to come," "to carry," "to bring") (Corominas, 1961) "re-brings."

According to these ideas, venous flux is one of the components of the innervation key of the normal process of remembering.[5] When memories are hampered, the key becomes deformed, and one component, in this case, the venous circulation, receives a more intense cathexis, displacing the importance of "re-feeling" or remembering to it. Consciousness then perceives an alteration in venous return whose "emotional" meaning is: certain memories must not "come" directly (by the shortest route).[6]

---

[3]The Hm memic trace is an information-structure, which, when cathected by an unconscious impulse, takes shape as an unconscious wish, that is, as ongoing information. This ongoing information may result in (a) repetition, (b) reminiscence, and (c) affective memories.

a. Re-petition (from "request": "to direct oneself to") is a re-action, a return to direct oneself (one's habits) toward an encounter with the object, which implies a discharge onto the external world (effective action). Repetition is predominantly hepatic, because the liver symbolizes the process of "realization."

b. Re-miniscence (deriving from "mind") is a re-presentation, a re-view, a re-minder, the return of an idea to the mind (idea: from *eidon*, "I saw"). Reminiscence is basically cerebral, since the brain is the organ that is mainly assigned the representation of the mind.

c. Affective memories, which are expressed by the Spanish word *recorder*, imply a return to the heart, to re-feel, to feel again an affect that involves a discharge on the body itself. Affective memories are essentially cardiac.

The prefix "re-" ("re-peat," "re-turn") means that repetition (re-action), re-miniscence (re-presentation) and affective memories (re-feeling), were "there before" as action, presentation (presence), and feeling and were dislodged by repression ("effort of dislodgment") or forgetting ("obliteration"). The prefix "re-" (in Spanish, the sound is "rrr") is perhaps linked to feelings of anger accompanying the current frustration. This anger-frustration cannot be quenched until the "original" psychical acts have been recovered, as a discharge in action (external world), in presentation (sensorial ideas) or in feeling (corporeal sensation).

[4]The important role of the vasomotor component in the expression of affect makes it especially apt for symbolizing all that is emotional.

[5]Obstfeld (1978) demonstrated the relation between the action of remembering (affective memories) and venous function, and between malfunctions of the latter and alterations in the former. The disorders of the venous circulation are related to problems having to do with the past.

[6]If the return blood reaching the heart symbolizes the process of remembering, we might well wonder what the meaning of the arterial blood that flows toward the tissues would be. We have not studied this subject, which is related to venous pathology. It is interesting to note that the "dis-heartening" of arterial blood coincides idiomatically in Italian with one of the forms of forgetting: *scordare*, "to remove things from the heart," unlike *dimenticare*, which means to "remove them" from the mind.

Varicose veins, with their characteristic signs, abnormal dilation of the veins, and stasis (remora) and reflux of blood,[7] represent a development that is equivalent to the attitude of delaying, arresting, or turning back the normal flow of some memories. Normally, painful memories are frequently delayed by avoiding perceptual stimuli that might trigger them. We must assume that the innervation key of this process involves a certain delay in venous circulation, within physiological limits.

As Foote (1969) reported, ancient documents state that varicose veins are dilations of the veins originating in a mixture of "black bile" (*melanos-colia*) and the melancholic temperament, since varicose veins can nearly always be observed in persons with this temperament. This description, linking the venous stasis (obstacle) to the biliary stasis (*melanoscolia*) and the melancholic temperament, led us to investigate the relation between varicose veins and cardiac melancholia, a variation of this disorder characterized by intense feelings of nostalgia, unlike the feeling of bitterness typical of hepatic melancholia.

From the metapsychological point of view, nostalgia and hope (*anhelo*), memory and desire, are the same process seen from different angles. We remember because we desire (or fear) something the memory refers to and because the object of our desire is not present. We then suffer from its absence and experience a feeling of nostalgia. Nostalgia always conceals a wish and, inversely, wishes always conceal nostalgia. Nostalgia (from the Greek *nostos*, meaning "return" and *algos* meaning "pain": "painful desire to return") (Corominas, 1961) takes shape as a "disease of absence," a pain due to what once was and is no longer, and seems to be specifically linked to the process of remembering (Chiozza, 1981).

In spite of the hidden nature of the feelings and the physical signs that become the key of nostalgia,[8] our investigations to date lead us to assume that venous function—which symbolizes the "return of memories to the heart"—is part of the innervation key of the feeling of nostalgia. In the cardiac variation of melancholia, the flow of memories

---

[7]Etymology indicates that the word "dilate" means "to extend," "to occupy more place in time and in space." It also refers to an operation of the mind that is "to defer," "to delay the arrival of something" (Real Academia Española, 1950). The remora is a "marine teleosteous fish" that adheres firmly to floating objects; the ancients attributed to it the ability to stop ships (Real Academia Española, 1950). Its presence on the hull of a ship slows its speed. The etymological root of "remora" (*morari*) gives origin to the designation of "a state of things: delay, detention, permanence," and also to an attribute: "remiss, loafer" (Corominas, 1961). The "stasis or delay" (in Spanish, *remora*) usually refers to the "stagnation of liquid blood" and to the "obstruction, detention or suspension of contents" (Real Academia Española, 1950), referring both to material elements as well as to ideas, emotions, or values. Thus, for example, we speak of a "stasis" in the flow of bile, in a country's economy, or in the economy of a person's libido. The word "reflux," contrary to "flux," meaning "advance," "progression," means "to turn back" (Real Academia Española, 1950).

[8]We can register the presence of the specific components of some affects. For example, the feeling of shame is usually accompanied by arterial vasodilation, which the subject experiences as a feeling of heat and the observer registers visually as blushing.

continues, accompanied by nostalgia.[9] The varicose disorder, however, originates in the destructuring of the process of remembering and of its characteristic affect, nostalgia. Varicose veins express and symbolize a development that is equivalent to the normal attitude of avoiding memories as well as access of nostalgia to consciousness, while fashioning another means of discharge from the same unconscious key. In this sense, the reflux and delay in venous circulation represent the attempt to remain fixated to the past and to delay the beginning of a process of mourning, in the triple sense of pain, renouncement, and re-signification of what once was and is no longer.[10] The contents of that "arrested memory" (remora) that "cannot" or "do not wish to" be activated, "to become" memories, are present in behavior anyway, tinging life through repetition.

The link between varicose veins and the avoidance of remembering and nostalgia has led us to discover another characteristic of the memory involved in this illness. We find that the difficulty in remembering means not only eluding the pain due to the absence of what is felt to be good and therefore desired (nostalgia). It can also include the attempt to impede the constant presence of a traumatic scene, which cannot be avoided and is attributed to the action of a "bad," "harmful" object. It is the "I don't even want to think about it . . ." for fear of re-experiencing the pain, of being trapped in the painful memory. It is the memory that is experienced as a condemnation, something that is repeated and cannot be escaped. It is the "torment of memories," which, like the eagle that visited the chained Prometheus, returns day after day.

The word "condemnation" comes from the Latin *condemnare* (from *cum*, "with" and *damnare*, "to hurt") and means "to judge the accused guilty, imposing the corresponding punishment or sanction" and also "to enter eternal punishment" (*Enciclopedia Salvat*, 1972). It is with this meaning of eternal punishment, rather than with the customary meaning of "condemnation" as guilt and punishment, that we characterize the feeling of condemnation inherent in some memories and implicit in the repetition compulsion. It is an experience impossible to escape: painful re-feeling in perpetual repetition: "It's always the same old story."

Nostalgia and condemnation are two aspects of memory that conceal and refer to each other. The pain caused by a certain absence (nostalgia) conceals and represents the current unsatisfied desire, experienced as a harmful presence (condemnation). Reciprocally, the fear that the current harm (condemnation) may become eternal conceals and represents the pain caused by a particular absence (nostalgia). Memory is united to repetition by the condemnation and to

---

[9]We think that nostalgia is an affect inherent to the process of remembering, regardless of the degree to which it has access to consciousness.

[10]In this sense the attitude of the varicose vein patient would be that of a lazy, indolent person who resists facing his feelings and starting an inevitable mourning process.

reminiscence by the nostalgia. Both nostalgia and condemnation are the first stage in a mourning process that ends when the renouncement to what has been lost "extinguishes the memories" and leads to re-signifying the present.

In line with these ideas, varicose veins symbolize the attempt to delay, place obstacles in the way of, or arrest "the return to the heart" of those memories that might set off unbearable feelings of nostalgia or of condemnation. In theory, it is possible that the particular content of the memories that remain obstructed or "arrested" (venous reflux or remora) is linked to the specific meaning belonging to the part of the body that is the site of the varicose veins.

B. Varicose Tortuousness

Another aspect of the varicose disorder is the particular shape the stricken veins acquire. Although in the initial stages they can take their course with a dilation of the trunk that preserves the vein's cylindrical structure, most authors consider the varicose veins a full-blown illness when part or all of their path is "tortuous," that is, twisted, sinuous.[11] The word "tortuous," from the Latin *tortus*, "to twist," is usually used to denote a "road that, instead of being direct, has detours, turns and roundabouts" (Real Academia Española, 1950). The tortuousness of varicose veins thus expresses and symbolizes the "detoured" road, full of "turns and roundabouts," that hinders direct access to unbearable memories. We find that the etymology of the word "varicose" contains the root *uar*, which means "detour"; from this, *uarix* (varicose) "detour of a normal vein" and *uarus*, "detour from what is straight, right and just, that is, twisted and tortuous" (Partridge, 1966).

Some patients suffering from varicose veins show us that their affects usually reach them, and others as well, in a twisted or indirect way. According to the Real Academia Española (1950), the term "tortuous," in the figurative sense, indicates a "way of being and acting that is characterized by beating around the bush and using indirect means in order to conceal a truth or to elude the difficulties of a situation." The tortuousness of varicose veins in the body can develop in a way that is equivalent to character development, in terms of difficulty in developing frank and direct expression of some affects, which consequently can be characterized as "the roundabout style." In this way, the subject attempts to "conceal" the affects that he/she feels are painful or censurable and to "elude" the difficulties felt to arise from more direct communication with others.

---

[11]Most of the authors consulted (Foote, 1969; Del Campo Llerena, 1984; Cigorraga, 1986, personal communication) indicate that the dilation of the vein does not in itself constitute the varicose disorder. Thus, for example, the so-called "athlete's veins" are thickened but are not varicose.

The tortuousness of the varicose vein, which, in its primary sense, represents the twisted road by which direct access to unbearable memories is avoided, also involves other fantasies of a secondary type. We find that the patient seems to interpret any deviation from his/her goals and values as something negative that must be avoided. In this sense, the vein's twisting course corporally symbolizes and represents those "detours and deviations" that the varicose patient cannot take in real life, that is, in behavior. However, the "crooked" road does not always mean error or immorality, as the varicose patient seems to believe. It also represents a stochastic[12] detour, which is positive because it enables a temporary turning aside from an objective that is difficult to reach. It is the linear nature of goals that often hinders the necessary detours that allow the person to reach the goal in the possible way, "finding the right turns" on the road.[13]

The term "tortuous" is also intimately linked to the word "torture," since both come from the same etymological root, *tortus*, "to twist."[14] In this sense, varicose tortuousness also seems to represent a state of suffering characterized by feeling "tortured" or "tormented." This "torture" refers to the difficulty in tolerating the painful delays associated with the indirect path (having to find roundabouts and detours in order to reach the goal). As we shall see, this meaning converges with that of the venous remora in the sense of the expression *hacerse mala sangre*, which means, literally, "to make bad blood" and as an idiomatic expression, "to get upset," "to harm oneself" (Moliner, 1986).

C. VENOUS BLOOD

Some authors hold that blood symbolizes diverse feelings such as love, hate, excitement, violence (Wyss, 1947), cruelty (derived from *cruor*, which means "bloodshed") (Ernout & Meillet, 1959), and so on. However, rather than one or several feelings in particular, blood seems to symbolize the passionate nature of the emotions (sanguine temperament). Bloodshed (both arterial and venous) is usually associated with the contents of drama or tragedy and lends itself to symbolizing the

---

[12]"Stochastic," from the Greek *stocazein*, "to shoot an arrow at a target," that is, to disperse events in an aleatory way, so that some reach the desired result. Bateson stated that a sequence of events is stochastic if it combines an aleatory component with a selective process, so that only certain results of the aleatory component are able to remain (Bateson, 1979). Along these lines, Chiozza (1981a) maintained that "every event in life is the product of a 'stochastic' process, that is, of the combination between an ego that tries to impose its invariant habits and the circumstances that condition an unexpected variation."

[13]A well-known experiment demonstrates that when a hungry dog is separated from a piece of meat by a fence that has an opening at one end, in order for the dog to "find the way," the distance between the meat and the opening must be shorter than when the dog is not so hungry.

[14]"Torture" means: (a) "deviation from the straight"; (b) pain, anxiety, great sorrow, or affliction; (c) "action of torment or torture," and so on (Real Academia Española, 1950).

passions. (Arterial blood, with its vivid red color and its capacity for "outbursts," for being "thrust out" by the heartbeat, could represent, even more specifically, the most intense primary emotions.)

Physiology teaches us that the main functions of venous blood are to collect all the waste substances left by tissue activity and to reflect everything that happens in the intimacy of the body, since alterations in the state of the organs usually imply an alteration in the quantity or composition of circulating blood (Wyss, 1947). Many of the laboratory tests that add to knowledge of the state of the organism make use of a small sample of venous blood. In line with these representations, Laborde et al. (1973) maintain that venous blood, which notifies us of the body's needs and disorders, symbolically functions as the "witness" that "demonstrates" the lack of whatever is "needed." Venous blood is "deficient or poorer" than arterial blood, since the latter has a higher oxygen concentration and is rich in nutrients. In this sense, venous blood itself "suffers" from the situations it "witnesses," just as a hungry messenger from a besieged city demonstrates in his person the want he is reporting. According to these ideas, the venous remora and reflux symbolize the attempt to avoid or to hinder the re-experiencing of those memories that conceal the present by referring to the past and at the same time bring "news" of present wants or needs that are being experienced painfully.

A patient we remember used to touch the varicose veins in her legs in an unconscious gesture whenever she spoke of having "made bad blood."[15] We believe that "making bad blood" is a particular type of upset or suffering[16] that goes beyond the "torture" represented by the tortuous path of the vein. When this suffering cannot enter consciousness as an affect, a remora or capillary stasis due to reflux sets in as its equivalent, leading to signs such as edema or tissue hypoxia.

D. THE VENOUS VALVES

Medicine considers insufficiency or atrophy of the venous valves to be the main cause of the reflux or remora typical of varicose veins. Many authors, however, maintain that it is the only cause. Although valves are not a component that is specific to the venous system, since they are found in other organs such as the heart, the general "valve" fantasy is part of the mosaic of fantasies that forms the varicose disorder. The word "valve" derives from the Latin *valva*, which means "door" (Corominas,

---

[15]Obstfeld (1978) maintained that varicose patients often use the expression "to make bad blood" and linked it, on the one hand, to the stasis of the blood and on the other, to resentment and a difficulty of forgiving. In interviews with varicose patients, Altman & Cattaneo (1978) observed that these people have experienced situations of great suffering and that they tend to "make bad blood."

[16]This would be connected to the expression, "to curdle/chill someone's blood," which refers, literally, to the thickening and stagnation of the blood.

1961). Figuratively, "to close the door" means "to make something impossible or very difficult." "To open the door," on the other hand, implies "giving reason, occasion or facility for doing something" (Real Academia Española, 1950).

Like the valves, the sphincters act as "doors" that open or close, allowing or impeding passage. Although the anatomical constitution of the sphincters and the valves differs—the former are muscle rings, whereas the latter are folds of endothelial tissue—the etymologies of these terms and the functions to which they refer—as "doors that open and close the way"—point to an aspect they have in common. The word "door" means both "opening used to enter and to exit" ("gate") and also "orifice" or "hole" (Skeat, 1882; Real Academia Española, 1950). In this sense, we can think of a more general "orifacial" function related to the body's "doors" or orifices; the valves as well as the sphincters can be regarded as particular expressions of this function.

The essential difference between the valve and the sphincter is that the sphincter "decides" in each particular case: it regulates the quantity of the flow, opens or closes the way, favoring flow or reflux. The valve, in contrast, "does not decide" but is programmed so that the contents pass in only one direction and are blocked in the opposite direction. The valve acts as an "opening door" when the venous blood flows toward the heart and as "a closing door" when the venous blood attempts to return to the tissues. The function of the valve is to keep circulation, i.e., the direction of the flow, in order. Valvular dystrophy "leaves the door open," producing circulatory disorder: there is simultaneous advance and return, centripetal and centrifugal direction, current and countercurrent in the venous flow (Lacour, 1981).

We associate valvular action in the circulatory apparatus with a type of order that is unlike the "cerebral" one, that of ideas, but like the "cardiac" one, described by the Spanish term *cordura*,[17] which refers to the health of the affects and determines the relative importance of meanings. Proper functioning of the venous valves corresponds to a state of order, concert, or "accord" among the differing degrees of importance of the emotions that are re-corded or remembered. Contrarily, venous valvular insufficiency represents a state of affective disorder, "disconcert," or discord.

The valvular patient seems to be trapped by unconscious sentiments with different meanings that "collide" with each other and is unable to develop affects in a more "significant" direction, subordinating or

---

[17]*Cordura* in Spanish is the noun form of *cuerdo*, the Spanish word for "in one's right mind." *Cuerdo* derives from "cord," from the Latin *cordatus*, which in turn takes its origin from *cor, cordis*, meaning "heart." *Cordatus* is the origin of the archaic "chordate." The "chordates" (from the Latin *chorda*, meaning "cord") are animals with a spinal cord or notochord (Corominas, 1961; *Enciclopedia Salvat*, 1972). Both "heart" and "cord" involve the idea of leading to the center, to "the heart" or to the main axis (spinal column).

renouncing the others. It is when this state of emotional disconcertedness cannot reach consciousness that venous disorder seems to develop as an organic equivalent.[18]

IV. Varicose Veins of the Lower Limbs:
An Approach to Some of Their Specific Meanings

Peripheral or superficial venous insufficiency of the lower limbs is extremely common. According to several authors, between 10% and 17% of the total population, mostly women, suffer from it.[19] Primary or idiopathic essential varicose veins are the most frequent (90%, compared to 9% of the symptomatic or secondary varicose veins) and develop in the second or third decade of life. When varicose veins develop in the fifth or sixth decade, they tend to be related to the changes brought about by menopause (Lacour, 1981). At the beginning, the clinical picture is predominantly functional (pre-varicose state) and its clinical manifestation is the syndrome of "heavy legs."

The most important functions of the lower limbs are: to enable walking, to bear the weight of the body, and to facilitate erect posture (Daniels, 1964). Psychoanalysis has explored the meaning of locomotion and of some of its alterations from its own point of view. In one of his clinical histories, Freud (Freud & Breuer, 1895d) investigated the unconscious meaning of the astasia-abasia of a hysterical patient. He interpreted Elisabeth von R.'s difficulties in walking as symbolizing "her difficulties in going through life," her "lack of autonomy," her "feeling of powerlessness to change anything in her situation," her experience of "lacking support" and of "not taking a step ahead."

Melanie Klein (1952) and later A. Aberastury (1971) contended that standing on two legs and walking figure importantly in the process of separation from the mother and are triggered by the intensification of depressive anxieties. At this stage, the child experiences the need to gain distance from his/her mother to preserve her from his/her own destructive fantasies, which he achieves through weaning [in Spanish, *destete*, "to lose the breast"]. At the same time, in weaning the child cannot help feeling rejected or snubbed [in Spanish, *despecho*,

---

[18]The cardiac valvular pathology may be related to the disconcertedness of those emotions that are yet unformed for the subject—that is, the proto-affects and the venous valvular pathology might be related to the disconcertedness of already formed affects.

[19]A pilot study in the Argentine city of Rosario (Odisio, 1979) determined that 45% of women over 18 years of age showed symptoms of venous insufficiency. We believe that the greater incidence of varicose veins in women's legs could be connected with (a) the fact that the girl's "approach" to her father involves a more complicated oedipal vicissitude than the boy's, and (b) the consideration, in accord with Freud's view (1933a), that the narcissistic erotic cathexis encompasses the woman's entire body, whereas the man's is concentrated in his penis. Women's legs thus acquire greater esthetic and erotic value and thus are more appropriate for representing conflicts in approaching the erotic object.

literally means "without the breast" and also "the feeling of being snubbed"]. At the same time he/she desires to "set out on his/her way" (*encaminarse*; the root of this word is *caminar*, "walk") toward the father. At this point the role of the father is to help the child in his/her process of separation from the mother and in the establishment of relationships with the external world (Aberastury and Salas, 1978).

Acquiring walking skills guarantees motion, which at the motor level represents the beginning of independence; at this stage, the child not only can approach objects but also can walk away from them. In this sense, the passage from crawling on all fours to standing on two legs enlarges the child's view of his/her surroundings, as well as the field of experience and the variety of possible actions. Therefore, the child's actions become more complex (Osterrieth, 1973). According to these ideas, the function of locomotion of the lower limbs symbolizes the movement or action of "setting out on one's way" or of "being bound for . . ." away from the mother toward the father, i.e., from the family environment to the outer world, with all the change and progress that entails.

The fact that varicose veins are in the legs seems to tint those memories that "must not return directly by the shortest way to the heart," which implies the specific meanings mentioned above: walking away from the mother toward the father and from the family toward the world. The varicose vein patient tends to cling to family patterns that keep him/her from facing a larger or more complex "reality." Advancing, exploring the world, and questioning values configured in infancy all seem to be too painful, too fearful for the patient and can become a source of conflict with those he/she loves. Various veins in the lower limbs often appear at turning points in life (adolescence, entry into adulthood, pregnancy, the onset of menopause, and the like) in which the struggle between the desire to stay the same, to go back, and to progress become much more intense.

Such conflicts are often related to hindrances in the realization of mourning. The pain caused by "the departure of what is over" is equivalent to the pain of "returning memories to the heart." Working through this process of mourning implies resignifying (an *a posteriori*, a deferred action of the affect nostalgia, which means a "painful desire to return and the impossibility of doing so") so that it may acquire a feeling of yearning in its original etymological sense, which used to be "hope," similar to the present Spanish word *anhelo* which means "a vehement desire of what is to come."

Therefore, varicose veins in the legs express a difficulty in taking a step ahead, in "setting out on one's way" toward another type of bond with objects and other stages in life. This feeling is specifically related to the attempt to postpone the re-sent(i)ment of memories, i.e. the feelings aroused once again by those memories, which among others, include resentment.

Lower limbs not only make possible physical movement toward or away from the erotic object: because of their anatomical closeness and connection to her genitalia, a woman's legs serve as perceptual surrogates for them; hence, the value placed upon their attractiveness (Morris, 1977). Varicose veins in the legs, which draw attention and at the same time may provoke rejection, symbolize the desire to avoid re-experiencing affects related to conflicts involved in approaching the erotic object.

A frequent sign, brown pigmentation,[20] a trophic skin disorder in the varicose clinical picture, seems to represent the signal of a desire experienced as a "stain" (something that would "tarnish the person's heritage or reputation") (*Enciclopedia Salvat*, 1972). The desire, although it should remain hidden, becomes "visible" on the skin—the return of the repressed.

As for the function of the lower limbs that enables erect posture, Freud (1930a) linked the acquisition of the upright posture to the repression of the instincts and the development of norms and values (culture) that became the guiding principles of human activity.

Most authors consulted maintain that a prolonged standing position tends to have a bearing on the varicose condition. The effort expended in defying the law of gravity for a long time, involved in certain professions and military duties, leads to anatomic consequences that have been demonstrated by venous angiographic studies. Prolonged standing—sometimes used as a method of torture—submits the body to a real torment. The expression "upstanding" describes a position that figuratively means "upright, straightforward." We associate this posture with a "stoic" character, a person who acts with integrity and constantly and firmly dominates his passions and sensitivity in favor of virtue (Ferrater Mora, 1954; *Enciclopedia Salvat*, 1972).[21] The attitude of being "upstanding" seems concordant with the problems of varicose patients who make an effort to "hold firmly" to their principles and to "be upright" in the face of affects or desires they feel are censurable.

V. SUMMARY OF VARICOSE VEINS AS SPECIFIC FANTASIES

1. Varicose veins are a pathologic alteration of the venous circulation. The venous system is specifically linked to the emotional aspect of remembering: "the return of the memories to the heart," that is, reliving or "re-feeling" affects referring to

---

[20]Pigmentation is related to the light-darkness cycle and to sexuality. Normally, hyperpigmentation is seen on the areas of the skin especially linked to sexual practices. Sexuality excites the melanocyte-stimulating system so that the sight of moles on the skin excites sexuality (Chiozza, 1986d).

[21]Stoicism is a very influential, predominantly moral and religious, philosophical position in Occidental thought. Its ethics are intellectualistic, producing a type of person who acts with integrity and dominates passions and sensitivity for the sake of virtue (Ferrater Mora, 1954; *Enciclopedia Salvat*, 1972).

the past. Therefore, we can say that we remember when the heart "re-feels" something that the vein "re-turns."

2. In the normal attitude of avoiding painful memories, there is a certain delay in venous circulation, within physiological limits. The venous disorder occurs when the normal attempt to delay memories becomes disorganized, the importance of the cathexis then falling mainly to the venous function.

Varicose veins, with their characteristic signs (abnormal dilation of the veins, blood remora, and reflux), seem to be the developmental equivalent of the attitude of delaying, arresting, or turning back the normal flow of some memories.

3. The process of remembering is accompanied by two painful feelings, independent of their degree of access to consciousness: the experience of nostalgia and the experience of condemnation.

The nostalgia takes shape as a pain due to the absence of what once was and is no longer. The condemnation involves the continued presence of an unavoidable, reiterative traumatic scene from which it seems impossible to break free. Varicose veins symbolize the attempt to arrest or to hinder the "return to the heart" of memories apt to set off unbearable feelings of nostalgia or of condemnation.

4. The reflux and remora of venous circulation represent the attempt to remain fixated to the past and to delay the initiation of a mourning process, which ends when the renouncement of what was lost "extinguishes the memories" and leads to resignifying the present.

5. The tortuousness of the venous path typical of varicose veins expresses and symbolizes the pathway that is replete with "turns and roundabouts," hindering direct access of unbearable memories.

An equivalent character development can be seen in those who have difficulty with frank and direct expression of some emotions, and who therefore "beat about the bush" (the "roundabout" character).

6. The tortuousness of the veins also symbolizes: (a) those "roundabouts and detours" that the varicose patient, for the sake of his "rectitude," cannot take in life, and (b) a feeling of "torture" or "torment" linked to the difficulty of tolerating the painful delay that the indirect route imposes on linear objectives.

7. To "make bad blood" gives shape to a particular vexation or suffering that goes beyond the torture implicit in the tortuous

path. When this suffering fails to reach consciousness, the venous remora develops as its equivalent.

8. The function of the venous valves is to maintain the direction of flow. Incorrect functioning of the valves, however, represents a state of emotional disorder, disconcertedness, or dis-cord.
9. In relation to the varicose veins of the lower limbs, we find that:
   a. The function of locomotion symbolizes the action or movement of "getting on the way" from the mother to the father or from the family setting to the outside world.

Varicose veins of the legs express the difficulty of "taking a step towards," of "setting out for" other relationships and other stages of life. This difficulty is specifically linked to the attempt to postpone the re-feeling of memories, a necessary part of the mourning process implicit in every situation of change.

   b. The lower limbs function as "routes" leading to the genitals; their participation in sexual attraction gives them esthetic value. In this way, they are able to symbolize conflicts connected with "approaching" the erotic object.
   c. A prolonged standing position, frequent in the varicose patient, can correspond to the attitude of "being upstanding" or firm in moral principles and unbending toward emotions or desires felt to be censurable.

VI. Case Material

JOHN

John gets back home late after dinner with Martha, his only daughter. His legs are tired and pained. Martha and Robert have just told him that they are going to get married, after having lived together for several years. Martha met Robert shortly before she divorced her former husband. He is an older man with grown children. There are some things about Robert that John doesn't like. Sometimes he suspects that he isn't very honest in his business dealings. . . . How different their lives are from his! . . . However, they aren't doing badly, and they seem to be happy. . . . What about him? He always considered himself an upright, faithful, respectful man; he never accepted the New Years' presents that some suppliers offered him when he was the purchasing manager of the hardware store. . . . In reality, he has nothing to complain about; he and his wife are happy, they lead a simple life and get along well.

John sits down on the bed, takes off his clothes and looks at the varicose veins in his legs. He had never paid much attention to them, but he has more and more cramps and pain at night. It's also hard for him to walk.

He remembers that the varicose veins set in when he was about thirty, after he married; now, at sixty-nine, he thinks that maybe they came on because he was always standing up. First when he was a young man, when he worked behind the counter in bars. Later, when he was twenty-five, an employee of a large hardware store, and then, when he set up his own store, with much sacrifice. . . . It seems an exaggeration, but he was always able to resist temptations. Maybe he was too honest to get very far. . . . Even when he was a kid, he was like that, respectful, obedient, he tried not to give his family reason for complaint, a family that was always praying and prohibiting.

He doesn't remember much about his childhood. . . . That big garden where they wouldn't let him play the games he wanted to play. . . . Dad, who was such a weak character. The image he had of him was of a weak man, who fought hard without achieving anything, who had happy moments, but was born to work and suffer. . . . Mom had to direct family life. With her he has a strong tie based on a deep understanding. His brothers called him a "snake in the grass" because he was always on her side, always said she was right and tried to please her. He managed to become the "simple, sensitive man, respectful of women" that his mother expected.

When Dad lost his right hand in the accident, hard times came on . . . the economic problems . . . Mom's health broken . . . Dad, who stole boxes from the factory where he worked! . . . He was only nine at the time. Sometimes stealing is justifiable. . . . That was when he turned into a tough kid . . . he didn't even cry when his father died!

He thought that marriage was something beautiful, but that it required great sacrifice and effort. More than once he rejected other women . . . was it because he always believed in fidelity or because he was afraid of falling in love? Why does he remember Margot from time to time? . . . She was French; one of the owners of the hardware store had brought her over from Paris. She fell in love with John and would go to him. He liked her very much; it was all very intense. She taught him the pleasure of dancing, of eating well, of riding on horseback . . . the things he experienced with her he never felt again with anybody, she was different! . . .

When she came back from one of her trips to France, Margot surprised him with a visit to the hardware store. How shocked he had felt! . . . in front of everybody! For them to see him with her, a woman who had been with other men! He had to leave her. . . . He did the right thing! . . . even though sexually they got along wonderfully. . . .

He had begun to go out with Eveline, an employee of the hardware store, a refined girl from a well-to-do family who accepted his mother's condition that they all live together, at least for the first year. When the year was over, they moved out so they could be alone . . . because Eveline couldn't stand it any longer.

A short time afterwards, Mom died. . . . Sometimes, he feels guilty for having gotten married and not having been with her more. . . . Luckily,

Eveline is optimistic, strong and energetic. . . . When they married he liked to give her French perfume . . . but some time ago his sense of smell changed, and now that perfume gives him a disagreeable feeling.

Things had gone pretty well for him in life . . . but now, since he came back from dinner, he feels down . . . with those varicose veins in the legs that hurt more and more. . . .

John constructed his life on the basis of a moral attitude that led him to block deep affects and needs. Since he was a child, he believed that he should grow up leading a righteous, "straight" life: being honest, faithful and obedient, both in work and in love. While he is working as an employee and then as the head of purchasing for the hardware store, he rejects any offer that might sway him from the "straight" road that he had set out for himself. Although he gets along wonderfully with Margot and is in love with her, he decides to leave her and marries Eveline, a girl from a good family with whom he could make a home.

Around the time of his marriage, the varicose veins begin to form in his legs; at that time, he must forget his relationship with Margot and separate from his mother, to whom he has a strong tie, based on a deep understanding. Leaving his childhood home to "go his own way" toward making his own family makes him feel afraid and intensely guilty.

John tries to postpone mourning for the loss of a yesterday he already feels cut off from. His varicose veins express and symbolize the attempt to delay the return to the heart of those memories that might bring on the pain of nostalgia for the loss of the close bond with his mother and of his passionate sexuality with Margot. Nostalgia that implies a condemnation: the presence of constant dissatisfaction in his work and in his love life with Eveline. The venous remora and reflux seem to represent his desire to "arrest" the memories, to "turn them back," impeding the re-feeling of the privation that is the perpetuation of his condemnation.

John seems to have accepted his mother's image of the world as if it were natural and unobjectionable: a world seen and judged by women, a world in which his father's weakness stressed the lack of a masculine point of view.

In Eveline he again finds the type of woman with which he is familiar and to which he is able to relate. In saying proudly that she is strong and energetic, he avoids re-experiencing his feelings of anger, submission, and sexual frustration. The French perfume, symbol of his love affair with Margot, has become a disagreeable stimulus for him that is able to evoke painful memories that he must avoid. Thus, only reminiscences of Margot, without their full emotional impact, reach him from time to time. Also, although he maintains that economically, things haven't gone badly for him, he avoids re-feeling his pain and anger for a business life that he feels doesn't reflect the effort and honesty he put into his life.

Apparently, John doesn't "make bad blood"; he seems to be content and without major conflicts. However, the suffering that fails to reach his consciousness as an affect "makes his blood bad" (the remora) and "deforms" his veins. His emotional disconcertedness, originating in the conflict between his honesty and his progress, or between fidelity and love, remains unconscious and is expressed in the disorder in his venous circulation.

The "rectitude" of his character is at variance with the "twisted" route of his veins. The tortuousness of his varicose veins represents in his body a development equivalent to what he is unable to achieve in his life, precisely because it was felt to be a detour or a turning away from the "straight" path.

The well-being of Martha and Robert, whose lives have been so different from his, reactivates the pain of his unconscious condemnation. That condemnation and that nostalgia, which remain repressed, are then expressed by the pain of his varicose veins.

5

PSYCHOANALYSIS
OF THE DIABETIC DISORDER

L. A. Chiozza, E. Obstfeld

> ... [A]nd that the thing had no solution.
> And inside, it bit me, tore me apart,
> corroded me, until the bitterness became
> a shameful, damned sweetness and
> finally, a great, undeniable pleasure. ...
> [F. Dostoievsky, *Notes from Under-
> ground*, p. 39]

I. Introduction

Weizsaecker (1950b) views illness with the idea that the physiological process in human beings behaves as if it were imbued with a psychologically comprehensible intention. In many papers, the result of our investigations into the different specific unconscious fantasies inherent to particular corporal representations, we have developed an approach to "psychosomatics" that transcends the mind–body dichotomy (Chiozza, 1963, 1970a, 1976). It is this line of thought on psychosomatic illness, originating in the ideas of Freud, Groddeck, and Weizsaecker, that guides us in our research on the specific psychical quality of the diabetic disorder.

In the case history of Elisabeth von R., Freud (Freud & Breuer, 1895d) stated that it is likely that somatic symptoms and language extract their materials from the same unconscious source. In developing his concepts concerning the erotogenic zones, Freud affirmed that any organ or important process contributes some component to the general excitation of the sexual instinct. He also asserted that from the goals of the drive we can deduce its source. These ideas prompted us to postulate that those cathexes take the form of representations or fantasies involving specific qualities emanating from the organs that are their sources (Chiozza, 1963). Thus, we justify, for example, the concept of hepatic fantasies (Chiozza, 1963), similar in theoretical structure to the oral fantasies widely accepted in psychoanalysis. Developments in the field of specific fantasies have enabled us to conceive, from a theoretical point of view, the existence of insulin-pancreatic fantasies. The drive components of these unconscious fantasies must possess a particular mode emanating from the unconscious source that is the insulin-pancreatic "zone."

In our experience, the patients we call diabetics precisely because they have something somatic in common (in spite of the singularity of each individual) also have something in common from the psychological point of view. We believe that the unconscious contains a common matrix from which, on the one hand, the material form that we know as diabetes takes shape and on the other, an insulin-pancreatic fantasy whose meaning bears specifically on the diabetic disorder.

II. Diabetes Mellitus

A. Brief Summary of the Literature Regarding the Psychodynamics of Diabetes

Menninger (1935) and Daniels (1936) mentioned the frequency of depression and anxiety in most diabetics. For these authors, there is no essential personality type in diabetic patients or typical mental disorder. Palmer (quoted by Miller de Paiva [1966]) was in accord with this opinion. Dunbar, Wolfe & Rioch (1936) described the personality of the diabetic, affirming that the patient with this disorder decompensates after a long period of tension and effort, has from infancy had difficulties involving indecision and insecurity, oscillating between dependency and independence, and is passive and masochistic.

Mirsky (quoted by Miller de Paiva [1966]) suggested that these patients' illness results from a flaw in psychophysiological adaptation to social trauma—that emotional stress is a trigger mechanism in an individual predisposed by constitutional factors. Meyer, Bollmeier, and Alexander of the Psychoanalytic Institute of Chicago (quoted by Miller de Paiva [1966]) emphasized that these are oral-aggressive patients with a contradictory tendency to reject the food and affection that they need. The outcome of this situation is an aggressive type of dependency on the mother. Diabetic patients have exaggerated needs for affection that are never satisfied, and their feelings of frustration are expressed in hostile reactions. Cremerius (1956) examined polyphagy, one of the symptoms of diabetes, and found that the illness becomes manifest when the instinct to eat no longer compensates for the subjacent neurotic conflict (paranoid, aggressive, and depressive states). Hinkle and Wolf (quoted by Miller de Paiva [1966]) found that diabetes is the product of a deficiency in adaptation due to physical and emotional insecurity which has developed in infancy, probably because of parental rejection when a sibling was born or because of the loss of the mother.

Newburgh and Camp (quoted by Miller de Paiva [1966]) concluded their investigations by asserting that there are emotional glucosurias. Meyer et al. (quoted by Miller de Paiva [1966]) described a case, treated psychologically, in which the resolution of the conflicts eliminated the need for diet and insulin.

B. Basic Concepts of the Pathophysiology and Clinical Picture of Diabetes

Current developments regarding the pathophysiology of diabetes are increasingly complex, mainly because of new knowledge of immune mechanisms and of the resistance of the cellular membrane. For our purposes, we will address only one aspect, on which all authors agree: that diabetes is an alteration of carbohydrate metabolism, due either to a deficit of insulin (usually a consequence of a dysfunction of the pancreatic islets of Langerhans) or to a disorder in its utilization. Since glucose cannot be incorporated into the cell, it remains in the blood in abnormally high quantities and is rendered useless as an energy source.

Normally, the level of sugar in the blood is kept constant because any decrease stimulates the disintegration of glycogen, which is obtained through conversion of glucose. Hormone factors, the most important of them being insulin, are mainly responsible for the regulation, production, storage, and use of sugar.

Insulin, in general, facilitates hypoglycemia-producing processes and specifically:

1. Favors phosphorylation and oxidation of glucose;
2. Contributes to the formation of glycogen in muscle and liver;
3. Lowers glycogenolysis (decomposition of glycogen);
4. Decreases glyconeogenesis (production of glycogen from fatty acids);
5. Facilitates the transformation of glucose into fatty acids.

For the purposes of our study, we shall discuss a physiopathological mechanism that we can summarize as follows: the diabetic organism suffers from insulin insufficiency, either because secretion is insufficient or because cell membranes are resistant to insulin. When a marked decrease in the tolerance for saccharides leads to hyperglycemia, as measured in the fasting state, the characteristic symptoms of diabetes become evident: polyuria, polydipsia, polyphagia, and weight loss. The complications of this syndrome comprise the consequences deriving from each symptom.

For example, the difficulty in assimilating glucose leads the diabetic's system to burn other substances (gluconeogenesis) in order to obtain the glucose necessary for survival and may lead to ketosis, which may be dangerous.

III. The Insulin-Pancreatic Fantasies

Although the psychical meaning of the metabolic functions is much further from consciousness than that of oral activities, we can use the representations provided by the pathophysiology of insulin in order to distinguish certain unconscious fantasies that we consider specific to the diabetic disorder and that necessarily have a bearing on the alteration of normal insulin-pancreatic fantasies pertinent to physiological saccharide metabolism. As we have said, insulin facilitates storage of glucose in the cells in the form of glycogen. Adenosine triphosphate, the body's energy reservoir, is a product of glucose metabolism. B. Houssay (1955) referred to glucose as "the mother substance of effort." In this process, insulin acts as an intermediary, facilitating phosphorylation of the glucose, which is thus converted into "useful" glucose (glucose-6-phosphate). In a figurative sense, the insulin "ignites" the glucose, just as a match ignites coal. We can assume, along these lines, that insulin-pancreatic function acquires in the unconscious the meaning of a representation of the disposition to expenditure of energy implicit in doing, undertaking, generating, or constructing. Lack of insulin, insulin resistance, or any other imbalance able to provoke a similar effect, impeding the diabetic from assimilating glucose into the tissues, would therefore mainly represent, unconsciously, a lack of the means for predisposition to the expenditure of energy necessary for doing work.

IV. The Innervation Key of the Affect Involved in Diabetes

Freud (1926d) asserted that the affect is equivalent to a universal and congenital hysterical attack, as the repetition of a motor activity that was appropriate at an earlier time. Each affect is a vegetative movement that is carried out in a characteristic way, a process of discharge whose "ultimate manifestations" are perceived by consciousness in a series that ranges from "somatic" feelings to sentiments that can be named. The quality of that discharge is phylogenetically determined by an unconscious mnemic trace, by a permanent register that Freud (1900a) called the "innervation key" that is part of the ideas that we attribute to what he called the "unrepressed unconscious" (Freud, 1915a). From the metapsychological viewpoint, "somatic" illness implies (Chiozza, 1974, 1976) that the cathexis is not displaced, as in neurosis, onto a substitute representation but rather takes place within the innervation key of the affects, so that some elements of the key receive a more intense cathexis than others. In other words, all somatic illnesses can be regarded as the decomposition of the innervation key of an affect during its discharge.

Normal metabolic functioning involves appropriate use of insulin and saccharides, and its unconscious meaning is necessarily associated with the feeling that whatever is achieved has been gotten by one's own means. Reiterated failure of that normal metabolic functioning is therefore associated with a particular negative version of the sentiment we have just described, which is that the goals achieved have been gotten by means other than one's own. This is a feeling that we can name the "feeling of impropriety." The etymology of "proper" (in Spanish "one's own") (Corominas, 1961) embraces two meanings, that of "proprietorship" and that of "appropriate"[1] for a particular subject, object, or purpose. For this reason, we consider this term especially suitable for naming the feeling that is affected in diabetic deficiency, since the most intense forms of that feeling affect the way these patients experience their own integrity and identity.

We know that a submissive attitude tends to inhibit the aggressor, even during fighting, in some species of animals; fighting usually centers on some type of property, be it food, territory, sexual object, or protection of the offspring. Therefore, from this point of view, submission is equivalent to recognition of impropriety. We can assume that the affect we call "submission" (manifesting weakness, formerly a motor act that was expedient for survival in certain situations), has a bearing on the feeling of impropriety regarding possessions (a feeling originating in lack of the means to obtain or to keep those possessions by fighting). We believe that a participant in that affect of submission, which from another angle is equivalent to the feeling of impropriety, is normally one of the innervations of its key: the inhibition of the assimilation of glucose, the main source of the energy involved in muscle action. Faced with an unbearable feeling of impropriety in relation to objects or positions acquired, diabetics unconsciously express and symbolize that feeling by hypercathecting one of the "normal" elements of their innervation key: inhibition of the process of glucose assimilation.

V. A PARTICULAR FORM OF MELANCHOLIA

The cells of diabetics are "impoverished and hungry" for glucose even as an excess of glucose circulates "uselessly" in their blood and cannot be assimilated because it cannot be phosphorylated. We consider this situation equivalent in a certain sense to that of "a pauper who seems to

---

[1]In Spanish we refer to the feeling as "*sentimiento de impropiedad*," meaning improper and implying "no property." The opposite feeling is "*sentimiento de propiedad*," which we translate as "feeling of ownership," referring to the feeling that we are the rightful owners of what we possess.

be rich," or who seems to have more than he does. We can also say that the characteristics of the substance involved, the "unassimilated" fictional wealth, linked to a denied feeling of impropriety, make diabetics dissatisfied people. They cannot make use of a "sweet" while, paradoxically, they cloy others and themselves.

To cloy is to cause distaste or disgust by supplying too much of something originally pleasant, especially something rich or sweet (*American Heritage Dictionary*, 1992). The wealth that diabetics cannot assimilate seems to be adequately represented by "self-cloying" with a delicacy that has been eaten in excess. Since the processes of metabolism and of identification derive from the same nucleus of unconscious meaning relating to the process of assimilation (Chiozza, 1970), we see that the metabolic difficulty also represents a deficit in the ego's capacity for identification.

We know that unrealized ideals can be felt to have been "lost" and may acquire the quality of a lethargic unconscious "object" (Cesio, 1960; Chiozza, 1963, 1970). This situation can be observed clinically as a special form of melancholia, with lethargic or hepatic (bitter) characteristics. Diabetics may suffer from a different type of melancholia that is "beyond bitterness," called "cloying" melancholia (Obstfeld, 1970). What we wish to stress is that in "cloying" melancholia the excess of "useless" unphosphorylated glucose unconsciously represents and also denies a particular "loss": the feeling of not deserving or being entitled to the means by which these patients live. According to Corominas (1961), "to become cloyed" probably evolved from the idea of being overinvolved in something and was derived from the word that means "to go too far out to sea" (in English, "to become saturated" would be comparable).

Freud (1910e) took examples from both the Egyptian and contemporary European languages to show that certain words may originally have had dual, antithetical meanings, and he suggests that at least initially, concepts could only arise through comparisons (although with further development it became possible to think of a concept without at the same time thinking of its contrary). In that situation, we may suppose that one of the antithetical meanings has become unconscious. Therefore, in the case of diabetics, we may suppose that the word "cloy" also refers to an attitude of "non-involvement," of "not getting into things," of not becoming deeply interested in the things they do. Weizsaecker (1950a) was referring to this attitude when he said that diabetics are neglectful in their lives and in their metabolism. This is clearer in the light of what we said about hepatic disorders (Chiozza, 1963), since diabetics are "beyond" bitterness, beyond envy, and also, for the same reason, beyond hope.

The word "diabetes" comes from the Greek *diabaino*, which is equivalent to "I cross, go through, pass." Its meaning coincides with the representations provided by pathophysiology, since the lack of metabolic integration of the glucose leads to the "loss" of this substance by way of the kidney (glucosuria). Therefore, we can say that in their metabolic disorder, diabetics act like victims of a particular form of melancholia, representing and also denying an act of unconscious submission in which they waste and squander what they need most. The inhibition of glucose assimilation, assigned to represent the feeling of impropriety unbearable for consciousness, is the nucleus of the specific diabetic fantasy; this nucleus is juxtaposed, like the skins of the onion, to the "squandering" of non-phosphorylated glucose (glucosuria) and is thus well suited to represent fictitious wealth associated with the deep-rooted feeling that satisfaction is impossible. The metabolic deficiency (cells "hungry" for glucose), which oral intake does not resolve (but can actually aggravate), appropriately represents that everlasting feeling of dissatisfaction. When squandering appears in diabetics' behavior as a reaction formation to an intimate unconscious feeling of not deserving or being entitled to the objects or positions they have acquired, they behave like the pauper who pretends to be rich, and their sweetened offerings, coming from pretended wealth that they do not experience as such, instead of "nourishing," only cloy.

Summarizing, we can say that, from one unconscious matrix, pertaining to the innervation key of the feeling of impropriety, the perception of the material form we know as diabetes penetrates to consciousness on the one hand while, on the other hand, linguistic expressions such as "sweet talk," referring to the specific unconscious fantasy of diabetes, originate in the same matrix.

VI. Some Character Traits of Diabetics

A. Rascovsky (1960) described some characteristics of the psyche of the fetus and postulated the possibility of regression during that period of development; however, since he also postulated the absence of frustration, he denied the existence of fixations in the fetus.

Freud (1916–1917), however, maintained that the concepts of regression and fixation are inseparable, since the subject facing important frustrations in later stages always regresses to a point of fixation determined by a traumatic situation during the primacy of a certain erotogenic zone. For these reasons, we postulated (Chiozza, 1963) the existence of fixations in the fetus.

We can conjecture that the function of the pancreatic "zone" in charge of the production of insulin is sufficiently important to be assigned the representation of a broader functional group in which it intervenes. This zone acquires, during part of embryonic-fetal development, a certain primacy, equal to a quantity of insulin-pancreatic fixation.

On analogy to the theoretical approach used to describe the hepatic character (Chiozza, 1963), we can posit that, depending on the degree of "permeability" of the ego in relation to the nucleus constituted by the quantity of insulin-pancreatic fixation, a certain diabetic character trait would be configured that can be included in other character formations. The weaker the coherent ego, the more it identifies with the contents of early fixations. When the equilibrium between the nucleus that contains the insulin-pancreatic fixation and the rest of the ego is broken, the character structure is altered, or physical symptoms that conscious perception identifies and groups under the name of diabetes may set in.

A person can have diabetic character traits without the corresponding "organic" suffering. As we have said, the symptoms occur along the "planes of splitting" of the de-structuring of the affects when bringing them to consciousness is unbearable. From this perspective, it can be said that regression activates a "pathosomatic nucleus" of the personality.

Meyer, Bollmeier, and Alexander (quoted by Miller de Paiva [1966]) as well as Cremerius (1956), among the authors we have quoted, referring to the predominantly oral structure of patients of this type, describe them as shy, inhibited, suspicious, indecisive people lacking self-confidence, inclined to self-accusation and to infantile attitudes. However, that oral character structure fails to explain the peculiarity of the diabetic disorder, since we also observe it in persons who are not diabetic or who have other pathologies.

The basic substrate of the diabetic character, in our opinion, is a particular form of melancholia that, unlike the classical type, is seen in attitudes we characterize by the term "squandering," associated with difficulty in enjoying things evidenced by constant dissatisfaction. The name "cloying melancholia" derives from a "syrupy" trait: by giving what the person "has" but actually does not "possess," he/she prevents repressed feelings of envy and hostility "beyond hepatic bitterness" from reaching the conscious mind (Obstfeld, 1970). Egotistical and stingy reactions as well as bragging and overprotection of those around them are character traits frequently observed in diabetics. We can assume that they are structured as reaction formations to identification with the "diabetic nucleus." The egotistical and stingy reactions can be interpreted as defenses against the feeling of "internal poverty" that pertains to direct identification with the meaning of the diabetic disorder. The bragging can be understood as a compulsive need to obtain exhibitionistic satisfactions, thus concealing "internal poverty."

Overprotection of the people close to them can come about as a consequence of projecting the needful, the "miser," the "pauper," onto others, while the subject pseudo-identifies with the "rich" and wished-for object. This overprotection usually takes the form of acts of guilt-inducing sacrifice that actually reflect repressed hostility.

VII. THE TRANSFERENTIAL RELATIONSHIP AND THE OBJECT IMAGO OF THE DIABETIC

During psychoanalytic treatment, diabetic patients or those with a diabetic character structure appear to be submissive, as if they were "soft and flabby"; irritation and uncomfortable feelings usually predominate in their therapists' countertransference reactions, along with intense feelings of guilt that are not always conscious. The therapist who fails to understand the unconscious roots of his/her feelings may become trapped in a concordant countertransference that induces him/her to feel "useless." Or, on the contrary, escaping from the concordant identification with the "poverty" corresponding to the insulin disorder, he/she may take the more frequent complementary attitude, identifying with the ideal and tending to offer useless surrogates instead of interpretations, like an overprotective and guilt-inducing mother, who produces submission, cloying, and lack.

Therapists analyzing these patients usually feel that the patient is never satisfied with the interpretations, even though he/she will frequently praise them. The hate arising from the dissatisfaction that the patient represses leads her or him, out of fear of reprisals, to attempt to soothe the psychoanalyst, "sweetening him up" with flattery and praise that cloy him and make him lethargic. If this "cloying" action also fails, the patient regresses to a state of lethargic resignation described by Weizsaecker (1950a).

Freud maintained that the ancient forms of the ego survive in the id and may acquire new life (especially in the initial phases of individual development); they are preserved as unconscious dispositions to the development of affects or disorders reactivated by regression. The different stages of embryonic-fetal development presumably represent phylogenetic evolution in ontogeny and thus enable us to use representations taken from the zoological scale in the attempt to conceptualize some aspects of the object imago of the hepatic patient and also of the relationship of the ego with that imago, on the hepatic level of development (Chiozza, 1963).

The analysis of myths, literary works, and linguistic usages, both during and outside the psychoanalytic session, confirms the spontaneous and unconscious use of modes of representation expressed by images of real or fantasied zoology. On the zoological scale, the liver begins to differentiate from the pancreas in gastropods. "Slugs," the gastropods of which we are thinking, are soft, covered with a viscous mucous membrane, and seem particularly appropriate for representing the object imago of diabetics who are often identified with that imago and tend to appear to be submissive and to give the impression of flabby softness.

VIII. An Example of the Diabetic Character

The humorist Dan Greenburg wrote a small book (1969) describing, with the sagacity of the ablest psychoanalyst, the universal character of the "Jewish mother," which we consider (Obstfeld, 1975) an excellent example of the diabetic character. Obviously, as the author explains, it is not necessary to be a mother, Jewish, or even a woman, to be a "Jewish mother." In one passage of the book, the "Jewish mother" gives her son two shirts and, when he is about to wear one of them, asks him with a pained and reproachful look on her face if he didn't like the other one. In this example, we again see the difference between classic melancholia and the variation we call "cloying." The two shirts symbolize a "double," abundant present, intended to produce great satisfaction, but the mother's question (originating apparently in the projection of her dissatisfaction onto her son) actually produces guilt feelings that provoke suffering, which can be interpreted as the real, repressed objective of the question accompanying the gift. In this way, the "overprotection" that seems to characterize the "sweetness" of the "Jewish mother" character conceals the "squandering" of, and "bragging" about pretended wealth and the intense unconscious hostility associated with the loss of a son who is growing up and becoming independent in his tastes.

The constant dissatisfaction so typical of the "Jewish mother" is also described by the author with respect to meals and the importance given them, mainly the bread symbolizing the diabetic appetite, the carbohydrate that cannot be assimilated. Bragging is also expressed by the persistent need to show off, triumphing over others, who must then shoulder the "hepatic" envy denied by the diabetic. It is important to point out, however, that this showing off is achieved through pseudo-identification with an ideal object (a child, for example) and that the ego therefore always suffers a loss. A "Jewish mother" "longs for" her children in whom she has placed all her ideals. The excess "sweetness" with which she represses her unconscious hostility toward her own hepatically unassimilable ideals, deposited in her closest relationships, and the guilt that she feels about the "sweetened" attack that makes her feel that they are lost forever, reinforce the "diabetic" feelings of constant dissatisfaction. They are evident in the hopelessness typical of "cloying" melancholia.

IX. The Myth of Tantalus in the Light of Insulin-pancreatic Fantasies

In Greek mythology, Tantalus was the son of Zeus and the sea-nymph Pluto. The myths telling of his crimes and of the punishments meted out to him have many variations. One version has it that in order to please the gods, he stewed the body of his son Pelops and served it to them at a banquet. Nobody except his wife Demeter, who was distraught over the abduction of her daughter Persephone, partook of the horrible delicacy. She ate the flesh from the left shoulder.

Tantalus was condemned to eternal torment, forever suffering hunger and thirst, submerged up to his chin in water beneath a tree laden with fruit. Whenever he wanted to take a drink, bending down to the water, it receded so that his lips never reached it. The fruit also escaped his hands whenever he wanted to pick it. Another variation of the myth tells how he stole the gods' nectar and ambrosia.

When we interpret the contents of this myth in the light of insulin-pancreatic fantasies, we see that the fruit, a "sweet" food in the first version and nectar and ambrosia in the second rendering, can be associated with the glucose the diabetic needs and cannot use. In the same way, the water in which he is submerged up to his chin and which he cannot drink can be interpreted as the unconscious symbol of loss of "water" (polyuria) and of insatiable thirst (polydipsia). Tantalus is condemned by the gods to suffer hunger. He has what he needs at hand but cannot make use of it. This drama of the myth, the true essence of his torment, seems to represent the inner meaning of the diabetic disorder.

Prometheus defied the gods in a way that enables us to understand his dispute as a hepatic drama which ends in the unleashing of his poisoned passion: envy (symbolized by Heracles' arrow killing the eagle sent by the enemy god) (Chiozza, 1974). Tantalus, however, was unable to attack the gods with the envy that freed Prometheus and submissively offered his own son, who represents his ideals, as a "sweet" delicacy. The cruelest aspect is symbolized by Demeter, who eats Pelops' shoulder, but the latent hostility was also expressed in the deception involved in offering the gods an "unwholesome" delicacy, this deception being the real reason for the punishment.

When we compare the myths of Prometheus and of Tantalus, we see a regressive evolution from the hepatic disorder to the diabetic disorder: in the first case, bitterness, envy, and defiance of the gods; in the second, the squandering of a "cloying" sweetness and the submission of a person unable to defend what is his own (symbolized by his son).

In structural terms, the drama of Tantalus is that because of his extremely weak ego, his superego becomes very persecutory and supportive of the death instinct. Unlike Prometheus, Tantalus cannot feel the bitterness that involves the hope implicit in envy. His "sweet" crime symbolizes the failed attempt to survive, an offering that is an act of submission; it fails because it provokes the loss of all his objects as well as his aspirations to ego integration. Whereas Prometheus steals the sacred fire from the gods in order to give it to mankind, a life-giving and creative action, Tantalus offers his son, masochistically renouncing

his own ideals in self-destructive action (Papaleo, 1975). Tantalus' attitude toward the gods in offering them his son represents the myth of
weakness (hepatic and diabetic) that perpetuates his submission and
powerlessness in relation to an extremely persecutory ideal with which
identification is impossible. Tantalus gladly[2] submits to a superego that
demands his own death (Garma, 1975). This situation is frequently observed in those diabetic patients who are characterized by self-neglect
in their metabolic disorder (Weizsaecker, 1950a).

In some variations of the myth, Tantalus is punished because he is
a thief, having stolen the golden mastiff that guarded Zeus' temple,
having abducted Ganymedes before Zeus appointed him his cup-bearer,
or having stolen the gods' nectar. These variations open up a richer vein
of interpretation. The golden mastiff represents the ideal, the nectar the
"sweet" food. Tantalus the thief of nectar is a universal mythic symbol
of the drama that diabetics enact in their body: they feel that they haven't
put their effort, their energy, into obtaining what they possess and therefore, they experience everything they have as not belonging to them.

X. THE "CLOYING" MOTHER IMAGO IN A FAIRY TALE: HANSEL AND GRETEL

The psychoanalytic examination of fairy tales reveals the regressive
unconscious fantasies they express. We know that the nature of these
stories is wish-fulfillment; this explains why children feel such pleasure
when they listen to them and why they insist on hearing them told time
and again in exactly the same way. But if we interpret these tales in the
same way we interpret dreams, their traumatic origin comes to light
(Garma, 1940), enabling us to infer that their repetition is a failed attempt to work through unconscious fantasies.

The tale of Hansel and Gretel involves two children whose family
is suffering great poverty. The stepmother persuades the father to abandon them in the forest. The first attempt fails thanks to Hansel's clever-
ness: he leaves a path of pebbles that guides the children back home.
Later, he is only able to leave bread crumbs, which the birds eat. The
children then find that they are lost and after a time come upon a little
house made of candy. Seduced by the sweets, they are tricked by the
witch who lives there. She invites them in and seizes them, planning to
fatten them up and then eat them. The story reminds us that the expression "to sweeten up" means to offer an attractive lure to the unwise in
order to harm and take advantage of them. This trap is not unlike what
happens in the diabetic's body. Hansel manages to fool the witch, whose
eyesight is poor, making her believe that they are not getting fat. When
she realizes the truth, the children are already strong enough to push her

[2]In Spanish, *con gusto* means "with taste," literally, or "with pleasure."

into the oven in which she was going to roast them. Thus, they recover their freedom and carry away the witch's gold, with which they are able, after finding their father, to escape their poverty.

The figure of the evil stepmother, representing a "filicidal" maternal abandonment, is equivalent to the loss of food (the state of poverty and the bread crumbs, which are carbohydrates). This situation, manically denied and converted into the "sweet house" that they eat, returns in the witch who tries to eat the hungry children. Both the stepmother and the witch represent the imago of the bad, "cloying" mother. The witch fattens them up in order to eat them, just as she cloyed them earlier in order to trap them. The happy ending in which the children deceive the witch and take her gold is a wish-fulfillment that covers up the traumatic origin: submission to a cloying mother imago that is supportive of the death instinct.

XI. Diabetes and Consumer Society

Diabetes mellitus is the third-leading cause of death worldwide (Serrantes & Cardonet, 1969). Each period of history has had its own predominant somatic disorders, which reminds us of the well known "fashion" issue in illnesses.

The psychoanalytic theory of identification enables us to find a nucleus of meaning shared by the nature of modern consumer society and the vicissitudes of the diabetic disorder. The introjection of an object, of a part or a quality of it, into the self does not necessarily imply an identification, according to Wisdom (1961). Identification necessarily means that the object included in the internal world must be assimilated into the ego and must be experienced as part of it. Wisdom stated that only then is the subject able to "see with the object's eyes" because the object is in reality no longer an object but part of the self. This is the essence of identification, the only process structuring a real identity. Wisdom considers identity based on the appropriation of the object's qualities by projective identification an illusory acquisition implying the loss of the object and, above all, the loss of the possibility of integrating it.

We believe that the self of the diabetic, beyond bitterness, does not incorporate the object but places an illusory identification in its place, determining a pseudo-identity that reinforces constant dissatisfaction and leads to hopelessness. Considering that the intense experience of rootlessness, the addictions, and some of the many social conflicts to which people today are exposed have some relation to difficulties in acquiring a feeling of identity, we can assume that there is also a point of contact with an unconscious hepatic and diabetic nucleus. An important component of the so-called consumer society is the dissatisfaction people suffer in it and their difficulty in enjoying what they have acquired, which stimulates the acquisition of more and more objects in an illusory search for well-being. The latter attitude always involves squandering, since these objects are not used and are for the same reason easily lost. That is, acquiring objects is in these cases manic behavior concealing a melancholic attitude characterized by a constant feeling of loss and dissatisfaction.

We could say that consumer society, encouraging acquisition "on credit," in which effort is deferred in accord with the well-known formula "enjoy now and pay later," again implies a difficulty in enjoying objects, based on the feeling of impropriety with respect to the means by which they have been acquired. A vicious circle is thus established in which they are usually replaced rapidly and continuously, "squandering" in the service of an illusory search for unattainable enjoyment.

XII. SUMMARY OF THE DIABETIC SPECIFIC FANTASY

The psychoanalytic investigation of the diabetic disorder has led us to the following conclusions:

1. The diabetic disorder and the group of fantasies that we consider specific to this disorder develop from the same unconscious source.
2. Normal glucose metabolism involves proper production and utilization of insulin. This process is specifically related to the feeling of ownership, which derives from feeling able to:
   a. Enjoy spending and saving
   b. Obtain and maintain, with one's own means, what one possesses.
3. Normal glucose metabolism is one of the elements of the innervation key of the feelings that we sum up in the expression "feeling of ownership." The feeling of not deserving or being entitled to one's property or means constitutes what we call the "feeling of impropriety."
4. We know that a submissive attitude tends to provoke inhibition of the aggressor in some species of animals, even during a fight; the fight usually centers on some property, be it food, territory, sexual object, or protection of the offspring. From this perspective, submission equals recognition of impropriety.

We can assume that the affect we call "submission" (a motor act that earlier in phylogeny was appropriate in dealing with a stronger party) corresponds to the feeling of impropriety regarding possessions (a feeling originating in the lack of means to obtain or to keep those possessions by fighting). A slight decrease in insulin activity in normal glucose metabolism is part of the innervation key of the submissiveness associated with a normal, conscious feeling of impropriety.

5. When the attitude of submissiveness implicit in the feeling of impropriety is withdrawn from consciousness, the diabetic disorder takes over its symbolic representation by means of a pathological defense that decomposes the innervation key (pathosomatic defense) and displaces its entire cathexis onto one of the elements of that key, decreased effectiveness of insulin.

6. A small increase in insulin activity in normal glucose metabolism is part of the innervation key of the attitude of affirming the feeling of ownership by one's own effort, an attitude produced as a reaction formation or as overcompensation for a denied feeling of impropriety.

The abnormal increase in insulin activity, converted into a hypoglycemic disorder, is understandable as a deformation of the innervation key of that attitude.

7. The concept of prenatal fixation points enables us to hypothesize an insulin-pancreatic fixation point which shapes an insulin-pancreatic nucleus of the personality; the extent of its importance depends on the intensity of the fixation.

8. The most evident traits of the character called diabetic are acquired, depending on the degree of permeability of the rest of the ego to this nucleus, through direct identification that copies the qualities of the nucleus into the character or through reaction formation.

9. Though all diabetics possess a diabetic character to some extent, not everyone evidencing a diabetic character suffers from diabetes mellitus.

In order to acquire diabetes, an attitude of submission must be kept unconscious, associated with a feeling of impropriety that is unbearable to the conscious mind; the destructuring of the corresponding innervation key must also overcathect the formerly normal decrease in insulin function.

10. The most typical traits of the diabetic character can be grouped according to those that correspond to:
   a. Direct identification with the nucleus of the insulin-pancreatic fixation, where poverty, unwise spending, stinginess, and inability to obtain normal advantage "exist." These traits are pusillanimity, squandering, and perpetual dissatisfaction;

b. Reaction formation to this fixation nucleus. These traits include bragging about pretended wealth, stinginess that fails to resist the impulse to squander, and a cloying, over-protective, guilt-provoking, and sacrificial sweetness that seeks to accumulate false merit and to provoke compassion in the attempt to diminish the feeling of having a debt the diabetic does not intend to pay.

XIII. Case Material—Bertha (Age 57)

Bertha was suffering from diabetes in which, despite medication, her blood sugar level reached 3.5 gm/100 ml. She was 53 when she began her analysis. She had been born into a wealthy Austrian family that emigrated to Argentina when she was 12. She studied in this country and became a lawyer. Her mother had set up an upholstering shop where her father worked. Her family was well-off although they lived without great luxury. She married a divorcée when she was already a lawyer at 34, and she and her husband had two children.

When Bertha was 44, her father died of a cardiovascular accident during a hypertensive crisis. At that time, she learned that she had in-herited money and possessions her father held in Austria and had never mentioned; he had always been stingy with her in money matters. When Bertha received the inheritance, she already was enjoying a prosperous life which her husband's efforts had made possible.

A few months after her father's death, she began to suffer from the first symptoms of her disorder. He had been slightly diabetic during her childhood. However, neither hereditary factors nor identification after her father's death explains why Bertha did not develop hypertension, gastroduodenal ulcer, or rheumatoid arthritis, that is, the illnesses from which her father suffered. Assuming that the unconscious "choice" of a certain illness has a meaning inherent in the drama shaped by the patient's biography, we must consider the father's death a trigger of Bertha's dia-betes that exerted its effects mainly because of its meaning and was only secondarily reinforced as the product of an identification. Identification alone would lack sufficient capacity for generating the physical alter-ation that shapes the disorder.

Taking into account that she was 12 when they came over from Austria and that her father visited his country of origin frequently, it is striking that she learned of the fortune she was to inherit only when she was 44. This leads us to think that whether or not her father withheld the information from her, Bertha, in an infantile attitude, did not wish to find out. Further, her husband's economic progress enabled her to live much better than her earnings as a lawyer would have permitted. Although she works long hours, her present job is badly paid and ungratifying, since she does her professional work in a state enterprise where she works mechanically without caring much about what she does. We therefore conclude that the inheritance was threatening to make conscious the intolerable feeling that her material well-being was not a product of her own effort. The money she inherited was deposited and became something "untouchable," not to be used. This inheritance is managed by her husband and Bertha shows no interest in knowing, for example, how and where it is invested. In this sense, her attitude toward money is similar to the one she had when she was a girl.

Bertha evidenced many of the traits of the diabetic character described above, such as indifference, constant dissatisfaction, difficulty in enjoying herself, and the attitudes of submission and sacrifice, squandering and overprotection toward her children and relatives, also reflected in philanthropic, but often ineffective, actions.

From her history, we learned that Bertha had those character traits long before the paternal inheritance intensified a feeling of impropriety toward her possessions that she is unable to bear consciously and set off her diabetes.

The following are fragments of one of her sessions: As she is entering the office, she says excitedly: "You know? I have the new car outside in the street. I'm afraid of not knowing how to drive it, that they might steal it! I left all the documents inside and I don't even know the license number. What if something happens?"

The fear of robbery is Bertha's way of representing in the future her current experience of loss and also of expressing a submissive attitude: she left the documents in the car, not knowing the license number. Thus, if it were stolen, she would have difficulty in reclaiming it. Her husband decided to purchase the car for her and also took care of everything involved in the purchase. Bertha only chose the model and color. Thus, she again found that she had acquired something without any effort on her part.

The non-phosphorylated glucose, which is useless for preparing to use energy (as well as the phosphorylated glucose made available by insulin injections), represents in her unconscious the possessions that Bertha does not acquire by her own means.

Reciprocally, the car that she has not bought and that she is afraid of losing represents, in the scenario of her daily life, that same disorder of her glucose metabolism. But "now," in the psychoanalytic session, the interpretations that she receives as a product of the analyst's work, for which Bertha does not feel responsible, become receptors for the transference of the unconscious meaning of the insulin disturbance so that when the patient communicates what is happening to her with the car, she is unconsciously referring to the type of relationship she establishes with those interpretations. When the feeling of impropriety "toward the car" was interpreted, the patient associated that in the evening she had to go out to dinner with her family, because her son had received the diploma for a course in social coordination. She said:

He feels it's something great, but I don't know what he's going to do with the diploma, because he's not a sociologist or anything, I don't know if he can work with that. It's that he's always been so afraid of examinations that he feels that having achieved this is something great. . . .

She adds: "It's a silly little course. I feel that way, that it's not an important diploma."

In this narration, her son represents herself, feeling she's always bluffing or deceiving because of her repressed feeling of impropriety; but she also projects these fantasies onto her analyst and, as if he were also bluffing, deprecates his interpretations: by belittling them; she "squanders" them as if they were non-phosphorylated glucose.

When the analyst's interpretation links the feeling of impropriety with respect to the car and what the son might feel about his diploma, the patient goes on to say:

> . . . I went to get the car, I never had a Ford. I have the feeling that my husband turned the responsibility over to me, although it isn't true, because at the beginning he had gone to see about it. To top it off, I have to fire the woman who takes care of my aunt. At the beginning she seemed very good, but she's useless, she hurts her, she's only interested in the money. I have to pay her and send her on her way.

Bertha is beginning to recognize the feelings of dependency and weakness associated with her feeling of impropriety a little bit. This enables her to show the beginning of her hostility toward the woman who takes care of her aunt, who represents the psychoanalyst, the object of her diabetic transference. It is a cloying object that disillusions her, "very good at the beginning," but later leaving her in want, as her father did by hiding his fortune from her and by being, she had felt, unnecessarily stingy.

At another point in the same session she says:

> What gets me is when everything comes all at once. Right now, I have so many things that I can't stand it. If they had come one at a time it wouldn't have been so bad. [Pause] If the car isn't there when I leave, I have to go to the police station to report it, right? [Laughing] Where is the nearest police station?

In her difficulty getting organized, Bertha is expressing the loss associated with the impossibility of using her own energy. Her laughter and the humor in her question about the police station reveal the manic character of her attitude toward that "loss": squandering.

When the analyst interprets the acceptance (submission) implicit in her attitude of leaving the documents in the car that she somehow feels is improper, she says, "Yes, the truth is that while I was driving here, I thought of how to solve this problem. . . . I thought that when I got out to come here, I would take all the documents out of the car. When I got here, I forgot, I didn't do it. . . ." Shortly afterwards, she adds: "What I like about this car is that it's red, it's the first time I've had a red car."

The psychoanalyst, as a product of his countertransference, at first felt flattered by the patient's words. He thought that the pleasure in the red car, referring to the color of his hair, represented appreciation for his interpretations; but he immediately suspected that Bertha might be deceiving him. Perhaps her fantasy of having "squandered" made her fear a retaliatory attitude and in that case she would have to flatter him, "cloying" him, "sweetening him up," in order to placate that presumed reaction. He also thought that his countertransference might concord with what Bertha felt: she had begun to like the car, but because of her diabetic conflict, not enough to be able to enjoy it.

Although she complained that she can't manage "so many things at a time," Bertha is progressing. Four years ago, when she began her psychoanalytic treatment, her blood glucose levels, in spite of the insulin injections, brought her dangerously close to the possibility of a diabetic coma. Currently, her medication has been reduced; however, her levels of glycemia remain around 0.80 gm/100 ml in the morning and 1.50 gm in the evening, with a fluctuation of not more than 0.50 gm. Her low morning level is sometimes evident in hypoglycemic symptoms.

If we had based our interpretations only on Bertha's narration and associations with respect to her childhood, interpreting the attitude of submission and the feeling of impropriety that remain repressed in her, would we have been able to decrease the severity of her insulin insufficiency? Perhaps we would, since the pathosomatic deformation of those repressed feelings is specific to the diabetic disorder. But we must further question whether we would also have been able to overcome all the transferential-countertransferential difficulties and understand the basic "meaning" of those particular feelings in Bertha's life if we had not worked with the knowledge of the meanings pertinent to, and inherent in, diabetic pathophysiology.

6

THE STRUCTURE AND FUNCTIONING OF BONES AS SPECIFIC FANTASIES

L. A. CHIOZZA, E. A. DAYEN, R. A. SALZMAN

I. SOME BASIC FACTS ABOUT BONES

A. ANATOMY AND HISTOLOGY

Bone, the anatomy's hard tissue, is a type of connective tissue that can function both as support (allowing insertion of muscle origins) and as protection for the "vital organs." The structural unit of bones is the lamella, composed of cells and intercellular matrix. The characteristic cells are osteoblasts, osteocytes, and osteoclasts. The function of the osteoblast is to synthesize the intercellular matrix, the collagenous fibers, and to secrete the alkaline phosphatase that promotes the precipitation of calcium salts. The osteocyte contributes to preserving the characteristics of the bone matrix by means of osteolysis and intervenes in the regulation of circulating calcium. The osteoclast resorbs the bone by digesting the organic matrix and dissolving calcium salts. The intercellular bone matrix is composed of an amorphous substance and collagenous fibers on which calcium salts are deposited.

There are two types of bone tissue: cancellous and compact. In the first type, the lamellae, one against the other, form trabeculae. In the second type, lamellae arranged concentrically around a central tube containing blood vessels and nerve fibers form the Havers system. These two types participate in different ways in the constitution of flat, short, and long bones. The cancellous type is formed earlier than compact bone, as discussed in the next section, and is transformed into the compact type by functional needs, that is, according to the biological principle that the organ's character is determined by its function. Compact bone

is characterized by greater concentration of bone lamellae, helicoid disposition of the collagenous fibers of those lamellae, and higher calcium
content. These characteristics give it greater resistance and hardness.
Thus, in its process of maturation, the bone hardens.

B. Embryology

Bone tissue is formed in two ways: membranous and endochondrial. In
the former, typical of flat bones, the bone tissue is formed directly in the
mesenchyma. In the latter, characteristic of long bones, a previously formed
cartilaginous matrix functions as a mold for the future bone. As a result of
the process of ossification, cancellous bone is formed, later resorbed, and
then gradually replaced by mature bone of the compact type. Around the
third month of intrauterine life, the primary centers of ossification begin
to develop in the median zones of the diaphysis; by birth, they are already
completely ossified. After birth, the secondary centers of ossification gradually develop in the epiphyses, the specific form varying with each type of
bone. During this phase, a cartilaginous disk (epiphyseal disk) remains,
which allows the bone to grow longitudinally. When it has reached its full
length, the epiphyseal disks disappear and the epiphyses become united
to the bone diaphysis. This process ends around age 25, when the upper
growth cartilages of the tibia and the fibula are sealed.

C. Bone Physiology

Ham-Leeson stated that bones "were created to solve the problem of
keeping cells alive inside a calcified intercellular substance" (Ham-
Leeson, 1963, p. 269). In bone structure, organic elements are associated with inorganic elements. The bone's collagenous fiber is resistant
to stretching, and calcium salts, because of their marble-like hardness,
withstand pressure very well. Furthermore, the close connection between
fibers and calcium prevents them from slipping apart, thus, making the
bone firm.

   Through unceasing processes of destruction and reconstruction,
bone is continually renewed. Since "old" bone becomes relatively fragile and breakable, its organic matrix must constantly be renewed. Bone
changes its shape constantly and reorganizes its trabeculae according
to the direction of the lines of force. In this way, bone is remodelled in
accordance with the weight, effort, and directional pressures it sustains,
thus maintaining appropriate resistance.

D. The Phylogenetic Evolution of Bone Tissue

All living beings possess some type of structure that functions as support and protection. Plant tissues, like the lignin of wood, function as

support and enable plants to counter the force of gravity. In lower animals (sponges, coelenterates, mollusks, crustaceans, insects, and arachnids), we find exoskeletons: hard support structures covering the animal.

The Echinodermata represent an intermediate point in evolution between forms having an exoskeleton and those with an internal skeleton. These animals have an internal skeleton formed of small calcareous plaques united by muscle and connective tissue. Although this structure makes Echinodermata more defenseless than animals with an exoskeleton, it enables them to reach a larger size and also permits insertion of strong muscles to facilitate movement.

Size and locomotion have influenced the structural organization of living beings. A large and heavy animal needs hard internal support for movement and preservation of its form. In the most primitive vertebrates, the segmented spinal column is cartilaginous. The substitution of bone for cartilage occurs in the bony fishes and coincided with their move from the ocean to fresh water. According to Weisz, this move and the necessary fight against the force of currents created a need for strong muscles (Weisz, 1971) and, naturally, for strong support allowing their insertion.

II. DEVELOPMENT OF THE CONCEPT OF SPECIFIC FANTASIES

We shall review a portion of the works of Freud that we have already discussed elsewhere (Chiozza, 1976):

1. Freud (Freud & Breuer, 1895d) referred to the conditions that determine the choice of the organ affected by hysteria and described the mechanism of symbolic conversion. When this mechanism functions, the choice is determined by a given organ's capacity for symbolic representation of a fantasy, which remains unconscious. He also affirmed that symbolic conversion can affect not only the organs of relational life—the hand or mouth—but also the organs of vegetative life, such as the heart or the digestive system.
2. He stated (1905d) that all organs can function as erotogenic zones and that (1924c) any relatively important process can contribute some component to the general excitation of the sexual instinct.
3. He pointed out (1915c) that the examination of instinctual aims allows us to deduce the organic sources of the drives and that every organ or part of the body takes on the global or general representation of all processes in which it is heavily involved.

4. We can deduce from what Freud asserted in 1920 (1920g, p. 57) that the psychical unconscious can be attributed to the simplest biological forms.[1]
5. Finally, Freud (Freud & Breuer, 1895d) indicated that both hysteria and language extract their materials from the same source.

Integrating these views, we deduced that

> Every structure or physical process is a somatic source for a qualitatively differentiated impulse. This impulse is also an appropriate and particular unconscious fantasy that is specific to that structure or process. . . . The physical structure or process and its specific unconscious fantasy are one and the same thing, seen from two different viewpoints. [Chiozza, 1980]

Since all that is "psychological is close to what the biology of our age has called 'interiorness'" (Portmann, 1954), we think that

> Considered as a "function of interiorness," everything we call body (involving form, function, development and disorder) is a fantasy: mostly unconscious, composed or structured from many "partial" manifestations or "elemental" specific fantasies, it can only be separated from the whole artificially. Just as the fantasy is a specific material reality of the body, bodily reality shapes a specific fantasy. [Chiozza, 1980]

III. The Destructuring of the Affects

We have said elsewhere (Chiozza, 1986) that the affect's characteristics situate it as a kind of "hinge" between the territories we call "psychical" and "somatic." On the one hand, it is a psychical, phylogenetic reminiscence and on the other hand a current, "real" somatic discharge. Every

---

[1]"The question arises here . . . whether we do right in ascribing to protista those characteristics alone which they actually exhibit, and whether it is correct to assume that forces and processes which become visible only in the higher organisms originated in those organisms for the first time. . . . The objection may be raised against [a view of reproduction that represents it as a part manifestation of growth] that it postulates the existence of life instincts already operating in the simplest organisms; for otherwise, conjugation . . . would be avoided. If, therefore, we are not to abandon the hypothesis of death instincts, we must suppose them to be associated from the very first with life instincts" (Freud, 1920g, p. 57).

Etcheverry maintains that "it seems likely that the tradition of Haeckel and that of the Philosophy of Nature are the binding context of the Freudian text" (Etcheverry, 1978, p. 56), and that "for Haeckel the primeval cell (protista) as well as the cells joined into a multicellular living being possess a soul" (Etcheverry, 1978, p. 37). He also asserts that "the equation established by Freud between psyche and soul is unequivocal" (Etcheverry, 1978, p. 36).

On the other hand, Freud states in his *Outline of Psychoanalysis* that the truly psychical is unconscious and that consciousness is an accessory quality added to only a few of these processes (Freud, 1940a, p. 158).

affect is: (1) a process of discharge involving certain innervations of motor discharges and (2) certain sensations, "perceptions of the discharges that have occurred and direct sensations of pleasure and displeasure" (Freud, 1916–1917). Freud (1900a) maintained that emotional discharge takes shape according to an innervation key situated in unconscious representations. The innervation key of the affect is therefore an unconscious idea that determines the particular quality of each of the diverse vegetative motor discharges characterizing the different affects. When an affect entirely preserves the coherence of its key, it is recognizable as an emotion.

Unlike neurosis and psychosis, which preserve the coherence of the affect, somatic illness involves its pathosomatic decomposition (Chiozza, 1976). The displacement of cathexis takes place "within" the innervation key itself so that some elements of this key are more intensely cathected than the rest. When the process of discharge takes place according to this "deformed" key, consciousness no longer interprets an emotional meaning but perceives a phenomenon called a somatic disease instead, precisely because the psychical quality of that phenomenon has thus remained unconscious.

IV. There Is a Bone Erotogenic Zone Represented by the Bone's Cellular Elements

Freud's concepts regarding the erotogenic zones (1905d, 1915c, 1924c), together with our postulates about each of the erotogenic zones, discussed in previous works (Chiozza, 1963, 1971), allow us to deduce the existence of a bone erotogenic zone whose drive representatives shape its specific unconscious fantasies. Therefore, the activity of the bone cells constitutes the erogeneity of that zone. In the process of bone formation we can differentiate two complementary phases: the one in which bone is generated, establishing its adult form in an ontogenetic developmental process, and the other in which resorbed bone tissue is regenerated. Two different types of bone have been described; they are distinguished according to whether the predominant function is support or protection. These functions, manifest in the existence of the "long" and the "flat" bones, determine variations in the process of ossification. In the formation of the long bones, we can differentiate three periods: (1) in the intrauterine period, the diaphyses are ossified; (2) during childhood, the epiphyses are ossified; and (3) at the end of the period of body growth, the diaphyso-epiphyseal junctures are "sealed." We consider that these three meaningful moments in bone development match three stages of libidinal development in which there is a relative primacy of the bone erotogenic zone. Further, the general concepts of psychoanalytic theory lead us to the conclusion that a disorder in any of those three stages of the libidinal development will establish a "bone" fixation point.

V. The Capacity for Support and Protection

The support and protection the bone provides to the body depend on a characteristic of the bone: hardness. As a corollary, we wish to determine what the ego's capacity for support and protection depends on. We shall examine the meaning and etymology of the words "bone" and "hardness," on the one hand, and on the other, of the terms "to support" and "to protect."

The Spanish word for "bone," *hueso*, derives from the Latin *os* and is applied figuratively to "whatever is central or essential in a person, discourse or writing" (Blanquez Fraile, 1960).[2] The Spanish word for "hard" comes from the Latin *durus* and perhaps from the Greek *douron*, "stick of wood." This is used to describe a body resistant to deformation and also means (figuratively) that it can bear up under fatigue, or is strong, robust, firm, and constant when undergoing stress. On the other hand, the Spanish verb for "to last," *durar*, also comes from *durus* and means: "to go on being, working, or serving" and also "to subsist, to remain" (Real Academia Española, 1950; Blanquez Fraile, 1960). The Spanish meanings of the term "to support" are: "to remain firm, to hold down"; figuratively, it means to "defend" a proposition; "to remain firm in a position without falling from it"; "to sustain," "to pay for the needs of a person, a family or an institution," "to give moral support"; it also means "to confront, to resist" (*Enciclopedia Salvat*, 1986). The term "to protect," which means "to help" (*Diccionario Enciclopédico Hispano-Americano*, 1912), derives from the Latin *protegere*. Its root, *tegere*, means "to cover" (Corominas, 1961), and a derivative is *tectum*, meaning "roof."

Evidently, the different meanings of the words we have studied clarify the relations among support, protection, and hardness. We can say that the capacity for support and protection depends on hardness, i.e., the capacity for resisting and remaining firm, for persisting. Considering the support and protection provided by the parents or society (which act from outside the subject), the superego (acting from within the subject but outside the ego, as a representative both of the id and of parental authority), and the character (which operates, in the individual, from the ego), we propose the following hypothesis: in the realm of psychological meanings, support and protection depend on the resistance to changes an adequate normative system offers.

Any system with the characteristic of resisting change could take on the representation of whatever tends to remain stable, persist, or last. However, lasting means more than just resisting change. A system opposing change can become rigid, fragile, and therefore not endure.

---

[2]In Spanish, "bone," aside from its literal sense, means figuratively "anything causing work or inconvenience" and also "something useless, cheap or of poor quality." It also means "the nastiest or dullest part of a job allotted to two or more persons" (*Diccionario Enciclopédico Hispano-Americano*, 1912).

Resistance to change alone is mere "chronicity" that ruins but is unable to harden. An adequate normative system is one that, in addition to opposing change, also allows for reform, for the necessary remodelling, i.e., establishment. "Stability" means permanence, firmness, security (Real Academia Española, 1950). Proper functioning of the "capacity for establishing" depends equally on the capacity to erect and to resist. From another viewpoint, we believe that an adequate normative system enables the ego to reconcile its multiple "vassalages."[3] This reconciliation requires both opposition and disposition to reform. The "capacity for establishing" is evidenced as stability and associated with a feeling of security. The word "security" comes from the Latin *securus*. *Securus* means "free of care, full of confidence and without fear" (Blanquez Fraile, 1960). Therefore, the term "security" refers to the capacity for taking care of oneself; its meaning is summarized by what we refer to as "supporting oneself" and "protecting oneself."

All actions tend toward change and at the same time must be supported by the resistance of a normative system that opposes change. In that incorporated normative system, the individual finds the support and protection that make up the feeling of security. The care that is practiced by the parents is evidenced as "security" once it has been incorporated. The term "security," according to its original meaning (*se-cura*), refers to the "presence of an internal" normative system, i.e., a supportive and protective ethic. Therefore, a feeling of security is possible when there is an adequate set of norms that establishes "the limit," that lends "support" and provides support for uncertain action and protection against harmful action.

The physical existence of a bone system that supports and protects and the "historical" existence of social norms warrants our thinking of "a single, common" unconscious fantasy of support and protection, linked to hardness, that can be evidenced in consciousness, from a "historical" viewpoint, as an adequate normative system and from a "physical" point of view, as a normal bone system.

VI. BONE TISSUE AND CHARACTER

Freud (1930a) stated that the formation of the superego relates to two fundamentally important facts: the human being's helplessness and prolonged dependency during childhood, and the Oedipus complex. When he referred to the genesis of moral conscience (the superego), he stressed that small children are amoral, lacking internal inhibitions against instinctual gratifications and depend on an external power, which is parental authority. This external authority, responsible for differentiating

---

[3]In *The Ego and the Id* (Freud, 1923b), Freud stated that the ego must serve three lords: the Id, the Superego, and reality.

the good from the bad, governs the children, granting them proof of love and punishments that imply the loss of that love. In adult life, anguish over loss of love may be experienced as "social anguish."

The internalization of the external authority, which installs the superego (moral conscience), is a basic change in human development. The superego is established by identification with the parental agency, an identification that is linked to the dissolution of the Oedipus complex. In this regard, Freud (1923b) pointed out that the child's superego is constructed according to the model of the parents' superego. Once this identification is achieved, the superego then observes, guides, and threatens the ego. At this stage, anguish over loss of love becomes anguish of moral conscience, which, according to Freud, is indispensable in social relations.

As to character, Freud (1933a) attributed it entirely to the ego and stated that it is formed as a set of prejudices (Freud, 1895b). It is created above all by

> the incorporation of the former parental agency as a super-ego, which is no doubt its most important and decisive portion, and, further, identifications with the two parents of the later period and with other influential figures, and similar identifications formed as precipitates of abandoned object-relations. [Freud, 1933a, p. 91]

To the previous factors of character formation, Freud added the reaction-formations, "which are never absent" and "which the ego acquires—to begin with in making its repressions and later, by a more normal method, when it rejects unwished-for instinctual impulses" (Freud, 1933a, p. 91). Ten years earlier, Freud (1923b) had emphasized that an individual's character adopts influences from the history of erotic object choices or defends itself from them to an extent that varies according to its endurance.

For W. Reich (1933), character is determined by repeated infantile experiences and consequently expresses the entire past. During psychoanalytic treatment, "neurotic character traits can be perceived as a compact defense mechanism opposing our therapeutic efforts." He postulated the existence of a genital character that is different from the neurotic character and maintained that every subject's character is a mixture of both types. For this author, character is "the ego's armor against the dangers that threaten from the external world and against the repressed internal impulses." It is worthwhile to clarify that although this idea of ego armor induces us to imagine the character as a structure enveloping the ego, to the contrary, the ego is character.

Reich believed that character is a chronic alteration of the ego, a hard structure that develops from the conflict between instinctual demands and the frustrating external world. It is armor that must be viewed as something mobile. "The degree of mobility of the character, the capacity for opening or closing up to a situation, is the difference between a healthy and a neurotic character structure" (Reich, 1933, p. 159).

Finally, Reich described the three processes involved in what he calls the hardening of the ego: (1) "identification with frustrating reality, especially with the principal person representing that reality. This process gives the armor its meaningful contents." (2) "The aggression mobilized against the frustrating person, which caused anxiety, is turned against the subject's own being. This process immobilizes most of the aggressive energy, blocking it and drawing it away from motor expression, thus creating the inhibiting aspect of character." (3) The ego builds up reaction formations against sexual impulses and uses the energy of these formations for setting these impulses aside. Whereas the norms of external authority imposed by parents or society and the "interiorized" superego norms (moral conscience), are experienced as foreign to the ego, the subject's own norms, incorporated and constituting character, are mostly unconscious and ego-syntonic.

The word "character" is defined as "the organic and dynamic group of an individual's basic characteristics, forming the structure of his personality and determining his behavior and attitudes," and also as the "sign that is printed, painted or sculpted on something" (*Enciclopédica Salvat*, 1986). Character is therefore a particular way of being that involves consistent and stable ways of thinking, feeling, and acting (ways that can be represented in a signal, sign, or badge, which becomes its emblem). That particular way depends on the habits and customs (system of norms) which the individual has acquired in the course of development. The sum of what Freud, discussing character-formation, calls adopting influences and defending oneself from them is what we call "the capacity for establishing," formed by a "capacity for erecting and another for resisting."

The health of the character structure or its degree of mobility depends on that "capacity for establishing." For this reason, we believe that it would be more appropriate to say that character is an alteration of the ego that becomes stable, and we restrict the term "chronic" that Reich uses to refer to sick, defective, or ruined character structures. We must explain that whereas Reich considers that it is identification with a person that forms character, we believe that it is identification with the statutes, the corpus of norms that the person represents. In this sense, we consider that institution, which is itself a constitution, is the process by which the statute is instituted, and that the process of institution depends on the "capacity for establishing."

If we bear in mind that: (1) bone tissue is characterized by its hardness, and hardness seems to represent constant order, a stable normative system; (2) the form of bone tissue is constantly being remodelled in accord with the pressures and tensions it must bear, the forces that act on the bone sculpting in it the vicissitudes of a "history," we can conclude that bone is appropriate for the symbolic representation of character.

VII. ORTHOPEDIA

Orthopedia has often been associated with education. Nicolas Andry, who has been credited with the invention of the term "orthopedia," was also the author of a treatise on the proper upbringing of children. The treatise is entitled "Orthopedia or the art of preventing and correcting deformities of the body in children by all the means available to their fathers, mothers and the persons who must educate them." In this work, written in 1741, the author discussed the problems associated with the child's development, including the psychological aspects. Andry (Del Sel, 1963, p. 11) symbolized the object of the new specialty in an engraving. It shows a tree with a twisted trunk that is tied to a prop. That is, the term "orthopedia" contains Andry's intuitive perception, in 1741, of the specific bone fantasy. The word "orthopedia" (from the Greek *orthos*, straight, and *paidos*, child) was inspired by two specialties that were taught at that time: calipedia (from the Greek *kalos*, "beautiful"), the "treatise for having beautiful children," and trophopedia (from the Greek *trophos*, "to nourish"), "the art of nourishing children" (Del Sel, 1963).

From the psychoanalytic viewpoint, many authors link education to the constitution of the superego and character. Our discussion above enables us to understand why education is linked, on the one hand, to the bone structure (by orthopedia), and on the other (by psychoanalysis), to character. The word "education" comes from the Latin *educo*, a term with two definitions: (1) "to raise, to feed, to take care of," and (2) "to make [something] come out, to take something out" (Blanquez Fraile, 1960). (As Ortega y Gasset wrote: the potato educates its sprouts.) The Spanish word *enseñar*, meaning "to teach," derived from the Latin *signa* (plural of signum), comes from *insignare*, which means "to mark, to designate" (Corominas, 1961). "To teach," according to the Real Academia Española (1950), is "to instruct, to indoctrinate, to give an example or lesson as experience and as a guide for subsequent action."

"To learn," as well as "to apprehend," derives from "to take hold of." "To take hold of," from the Latin *prehendere*, means "to take, to trap, to surprise." According to the Real Academia Española (1950), "to learn" has three meanings: (1) to acquire knowledge of something by study or experience; (2) to conceive of something only by its appearance or with little basis; and (3) to take something into the memory. "To understand," also deriving from *prehendere*, means: (1) to embrace, to surround something completely; (2) to contain, to include in oneself;

and (3) to understand, to reach, to penetrate. A tolerant person, tendency, or attitude is "understanding."

The term "to discipline," according to the Real Academia Española (1950), has three definitions: (1) to instruct, to teach someone his profession by giving him lessons; (2) to impose, to enforce discipline, observance of the laws, on a person; (3) to beat, to whip with a cane as mortification or punishment.

Corominas (1961) pointed out that the word "doctor," from the Latin *doctororis* (master, one who teaches), comes from *docere* ("to teach"). In turn, *docto*, "wise," *doctus*, "learned," *docilis*, "who learns easily," and *documentum*, "teaching, example, sample" derive from the same term. "Docile," therefore, refers to one who learns easily and "docility," to aptitude for learning.

The etymology and semantics of "education" lead us to conclude that education integrates undeveloped aspects into the ego, aspects that in psychoanalysis we call "unborn aspects." Our text will refer to the original meaning of the word "education," "leading outward" and not the common definition, which is much broader. In order to integrate the "unborn aspects," education uses teaching and discipline. Teaching "gives (shows, points out) an example," while discipline (the canings) "breaks the shell" of character that impedes the birth of these aspects. In this view, education, the process which institutes the set of statutes that form character, begins by teaching and, through learning in a framework of discipline, reaches the understanding that makes the new norm into "bone." Docility thus permits the individual to learn from the master's example and to become what is called "an example."

But this process of institution (instruction)[4] can be disturbed, as sometimes happens in the process of identification. Both lack of docility and chronic docility hinder learning. In these cases, the individual can only "follow the example" and is unable to become an "accomplished example."

VIII. The Protection Barrier Against Stimuli: The Function of Calcium and Character

In "Beyond the pleasure principle" (1920g), Freud described the simplest possible living organism as an undifferentiated vesicle of excitable substance. This description enabled him to interrelate the genesis of consciousness, the location of the conscious system, and the peculiarities of the excitatory process of the latter system. He indicated that this particle of living substance would be annihilated by the balancing,

---

[4]The term "to instruct" derives from the Latin *instruo*. *Struo* means "to stack, to accumulate, to pile up." The word "to institute" derives from the Latin *in-statuo*. *Statuo* means "to erect." As the origins of the terms demonstrate, "to instruct" and "to institute" refer to the process by which something is "constituted."

and therefore, destructive influence of the energy of the "external" world if it lacked "protection against stimuli." Its surface therefore loses the structure of living matter and becomes "inorganic." Because of that protection, only a fraction of the intensity of the stimuli spreads to the contiguous layers, which receive stimuli that have been "filtered." Later, Freud affirmed that the psyche tends to treat internal excitations that cause an excessive multiplication of displeasure as if they originated not within but from without, in order to apply the same means of defense against them. He also suggested that we call those external excitations that are forceful enough to perforate the barrier against stimuli "traumatic."

Physiology uses a model very similar to Freud's to explain the function of calcium in triggering the action potential of the membrane, a process by which the transmission of the nerve stimulus is inhibited. It is important to remember that the bone apparatus, in addition to accomplishing its mission of support and protection, is the warehouse for the calcium that enters the blood stream (when necessary) to operate on the membrane, performing a function (inhibition) that we consider (from the psychoanalytic point of view) a "protective barrier against stimuli."[5] Reich's model for describing character-formation is remarkably similar to that of this barrier. He wrote that

> In the ego, character is formed in the part of the personality exposed to the external world; it is a sort of buffer in the struggle between the id and the external world. . . . Among these primitive needs on the one hand and the external world on the other, the ego gradually develops by differentiating itself from part of the psyche. This differentiation of part of the psyche reminds us of certain protozoans that protect themselves against the external world with a shield or shell of inorganic matter. . . . In the same way, the ego's character can be conceived as the shield that protects the id from the action of the external world. . . . Although the main reason for character-formation was protection from the external world, this is not its main function later. . . . The protection-mechanisms

---

[5]Guyton (1971) stated that

> The excess of calcium ions in the extracellular fluid reduces the permeability of the nerve membrane to sodium. The calcium ions also have a high potential for protein fixation. Therefore, it is believed that in normal conditions, the walls of sodium ducts—whatever these may be: pores, protein molecules scattered throughout a membrane, etc.—are lined with calcium ions. Because of their positive charges, the calcium ions repel sodium and other positive ions and hinder their passage through the ducts. [p. 60] When the concentration of calcium ions in the extra-cellular fluid falls below normal, the nervous system becomes more excitable, perhaps because of the increased permeability of the membranes. . . . When the level of calcium in the body rises above normal, the nervous system is inhibited and the reflex activity of the central nervous system diminishes. Also the muscles become lazy and weak, probably as a result of the effect of calcium on the muscle cell membranes. [p. 982]

of the character typically enter into action when there is a threat of danger from inside, from an instinctive impulse. Then, it is the task of the character to dominate anxiety caused by the energies of the impulses whose expression is made impossible.

IX. The Pathosomatic Deformation of the Specific Affects of Bone Function

Freud's ideas, statements in the field of physiology, and Reich's concepts allow us to identify the specific affects represented by the functions and disorders of the bones. We wish to return now to Freud's suggestion that we call traumatic those external excitations forceful enough to perforate the barrier against stimuli. Elsewhere (Chiozza, 1963, p. 208), we remarked that "If the ego cannot defend itself from a stimulus or a disproportionate impression (being 'impressed'), we find ourselves in the traumatic situation described by Garma (1956), who considers that dreams, 'beyond the pleasure principle,' are precisely hallucinations provoked by this type of traumatic situation." In our theory, this situation is the equivalent of

> the dissociation of the ego and the formation of a visual-ideal nucleus, at the expense of what was the ego's visual-ideal pole or zone. The traumatic situation is damage already inflicted on the psyche involving some disorganization. . . . If the stimulus disorganizes part of the ego and the rest defends itself by dissociating, the dissociated part containing the stimulus that must be bound anabolically, constitutes an "internal protopersecutor." [Chiozza, 1963, pp. 239–240]

Using a model similar to the one above, we deduce that when the ego is unable to defend itself from a stimulus that goes beyond its capacity for remodelling, for reforming its normative system or "capacity for establishing," then a traumatic situation results. We believe that the degree of health of a character structure depends on its capacity to remodel the normative system.

The traumatic situation implies a dissociation of the ego. When it faces the need to remodel a normative system that is anachronistic and therefore weak, three outcomes are possible: the experience of "falling to pieces," that of "infraction," or that of "consolidation." When any of these affects becomes unbearable to consciousness and there is pathosomatic deformation, a bone disorder may become manifest as a product of the hypercathexis of one of the elements of the key of the affect in question.

Destruction of the architecture and diminution of the bone mass, as in osteoporosis or osteomyelitis, in which the subject seems to "crumble," can be a melancholic variation of the "bone" disease. In these conditions the feeling of "falling to pieces" is realized symbolically by the bone disorder representing it.

The fracture is a manic variation that can be viewed as an attack on the supportive, protective bone when it is "confused" with the rigid normative system that is impossible to remodel. In such circumstances, the attack acquires the nature of an infraction which becomes unbearable to consciousness. The term "infraction," according to Corominas (1961), comes from the Latin *infringo*, "to break, to beat down, to interrupt the harmony," which in turns derives from *frangere*, "to break." Another derivative of *frangere* is the word "fracture." Therefore, the fracture represents a manic attempt to break a law and the denial of the feeling of infraction expressed by the prefix *in-*.

The increase in osteoblast activity that leads to hyperostosis (increase in bone density), as in Paget's disease, is a paranoid variation, in which the persecutor is represented by a remodelling influence that must be resisted. (The "minor forms" of hyperostosis, such as exostoses on different bones, e.g., osteophytes on the vertebrae, are quite frequent.) The consolidation of a normative system always involves the confirmation of an alliance and docility in adopting an influence. One of the definitions of the term "to consolidate," according to the Real Academia Española (1950), is "to unite the attributes of a previously disaggregated dominion in one subject." At times the docility implicit in consolidation remains unconscious and that only the desire to resist the influence of a former erotic object choice is consciously experienced. In this case, if consolidation of the normative system becomes intolerable to the conscious mind, then the confirmation of the system, represented by the bone, is expressed by hyperostosis.

X. The Feeling of Falling to Pieces: Infraction and Consolidation as They Relate to Solidity and Solidarity

Bodies having more cohesive molecules than those of liquids are called "solids." In the event of an impact that tends to disorganize them, their greater cohesion enables them to resist deformation through the degree of molecular cohesion, or "solidarity," among the constituent parts. As we know, "bone" is one of the most solid and hardest parts of an animal's body. According to the dictionary of etymology (Corominas, 1961), the word "solid" derives from the Latin term *solidus*, which means "firm, consistent." *Solidamentum*, which in Latin means "frame of the human body, skeleton," comes from the Latin *solidare*, which means "to solder, to strengthen, to harden." *Solidare* also means "to join the broken bones" and "to ratify." The word *solidarietas*, from late Latin, apparently introduced by the Church, is used to refer to solidarity (Blanquez Fraile, 1960).

The law uses the expression *in solidum*, meaning "by the whole," to refer to a type of obligation in common. Such an obligation is characterized by the fact that creditors can sue any one of the creditors for its entire value.

Christianity recognizes solidarity in the fact that each of the members responds for the whole group. For example, Christ gives his life for others. Solidarity is linked to a situation of reciprocal need between the members.

From a philosophical perspective, solidarity is

> the affective or emotional expression of our social condition. . . . It is a kind of individual and social sinovia [synovial fluid]. . . . The individual is solidary with himself, since he is internally a society. When the agglutinating factor of solidarity is lacking, the individual becomes unbalanced and the society disorganized. . . . Education, traditions, the social medium in which we move like the atmosphere that nourishes us . . . the examples we have received, in sum, all the ballast and sediment of public custom and opinion determine habits . . . that represent an extraordinary force that gravitates on the personal agent and sometimes exercises a kind of moral coercion. [*Diccionario Enciclopédico Hispano-Americano*, 1912]

Solidarity is characteristic of all solid bodies, be they bodies from the physical viewpoint or solidly united social bodies. In a relationship, solidarity[6] implies that each of the associated parts obtains some advantage from life in common and that all are equally responsible for the maintenance of the relationship and for its consequences. The modes of relating in a relationship characterized by solidarity are based on the healthiest character traits. The most rigid traits, less susceptible of reform, produce adhesive relationships which lack solidarity. Therefore, they are symbiotic relationships sustained by anachronistic habits and customs experienced as impossible to reform. This experience arises from the fact that these habits defend the ego from the integration of unborn aspects. These aspects, projected on a partner, are manifest in adhesion to a symbiotic relationship unable to develop the solidarity of a genital relationship.

When the development of the relationship requires a reform of the character trait expressed by the adhesion, this need for reform is experienced as an upheaval provoking the feeling of falling to pieces, of infraction or consolidation. These affects thus signal the disturbance of a habit or a way of being that prevents the birth of an unborn aspect of the ego and leads to establishing adhesive bonds lacking in solidarity.

---

[6]Spanish has a noun, *solidaridad*, that conveys the idea of solidarity, as well as words to express adjectival and verbal forms of this meaning. English, so far as we know, lacks equivalent forms.

XI. Summary of the Specific Bone Fantasy

1. There is an unconscious fantasy of support and protection, linked to hardness, that can reach consciousness, from a "psychical" viewpoint, as a feeling of security and from a "physical" viewpoint, as a normal bone apparatus.

2. The feeling of security ("security" derives from *se-cu-ra*, which means "to take care of oneself") arises when the care, exercised at first by the parents, is constituted as a function of the ego by a process that delegates it to an intermediary stage, the superego.

3. This care, exercised as support and protection, is established as ethics, a normative system instituted or constituted in the character as stable statutes throughout a process of education and learning.

4. Education, according to its original meaning, leads toward the outside, develops the "unborn aspects of the ego," using learning, which draws on the necessary elements from the outside. Both are facilitated by teaching, which shows, gives an example, indicates, or signals, and by discipline, which corrects, destroys, or modifies in the manner of tutelage or orthopedia.

5. A healthy or adequate normative system is one that, in addition to lending itself to reform, the remodelling necessary for creating new statutes as a product of the changes involved in education or learning, is also capable of opposing those changes by a certain amount of "inertia" or resistance.

6. The capacity for establishing a healthy normative statute therefore consists of an adequate proportion of the capacity for erecting on the one hand and the capacity for resisting on the other—in Freud's terms, for adopting the influences arising from the history of choices of erotic objects and for defending oneself against such influences.

7. Its hardness and capacity for remodelling itself according to varying degrees of stress, traction, and pressure that changes of function impose upon it are the most characteristic properties of bone. The "idea" that forms its structure corresponds to the "ingenuity" of a substance that keeps itself alive, immersed in a calcified environment possessing an essential property resembling inert matter: hardness.

8. The solid body that resists deformation through solidarity of its constituent parts with the part that suffers an impact is "hard" (in the figurative sense, someone who can withstand fatigue and is strong, robust and firm in the face of adversity). To last is also to subsist, to remain.

9. Because of its hardness, the bone gives support (sustenance, resistance, and firmness) and protection (shelter). The long bones are the outstanding representatives of the former function, whereas the flat bones represent the latter.

10. Bone tissue, because of its capacity for remodelling and characteristic hardness, can therefore be assigned the representation of the

THE STRUCTURE AND FUNCTIONING OF BONES AS SPECIFIC FANTASIES

establishment of an "internal" normative system or of the normative system itself in any of its forms: parents, teachers, society, the super-ego, or the character.

11. Three meaningful moments in bone development (intrauter-ine, childhood, and the termination of body growth) that match three periods in which the greatest changes in the normative system should occur also match, in terms of libidinal development, three phases of a relative primacy of the bone erotogenic zone. A disorder in any of these three stages of libidinal development establishes a "bone" fixation point.

12. Since the feeling of security derives from the adequate func-tioning of a normative system that gives support and protection, and since the structure and functioning of the bones take on the represen-tation of this system, we conclude that the normal functioning of bone tissue must necessarily be part of the innervation key of the feeling of security.

13. When an individual needs to remodel a malfunctioning normative system, he/she can experience three different affects: the feeling of falling to pieces, of infraction, or of consolidation. When consciousness cannot bear these feelings and their pathosomatic de-formation occurs, a bone disorder can arise as a result of a discharge that has occurred as a result of the hypercathexis of one of the elements of its key.

14. Destruction of bone architecture and the reduction in bone mass, as in osteoporosis or in osteomyelitis, is a melancholic varia-tion of "bone" disease. In such disorders, the feeling of falling to pieces is realized symbolically through the bone disorder that repre-sents it.

15. The fracture, a manic variation, can be viewed as an attack on the bone that supports and protects, when it is "mistaken" for a rigid normative system that is impossible to remodel. In these conditions, the attack acquires the nature of an infraction and becomes unbearable to consciousness. The fracture therefore represents a manic attempt to break a law and the denial of the feeling of infraction.

16. The increase in osteoblast activity that leads to hyperostosis is a paranoid variation in which the persecutor is represented by a re-modelling influence that must be resisted. The consolidation of a nor-mative system always involves the affirmation of an alliance and of docility for adopting an influence. It can happen that the docility involved in consolidation remains unconscious and only the desire to resist the adoption of the influence provided by the history of an erotic object choice becomes known. In this case, when the consoli-dation of the normative system becomes unbearable to consciousness, ratification of the system, represented by the bone, is expressed by hyperostosis.

XII. Case Material—Frank (age 70)

Suddenly, light. Sounds of buckets, metal furniture scraping and banging. The maids talking loudly, not caring in the least, as if they were alone. And he, who was barely able to sleep. All night thinking. . . .

The mornings are always the same. . . . At five the racket starts. Every morning. . . . It's been a year and a half now. It makes him so mad, but he has to keep calm.

When he was hospitalized, he thought it would only be for a few days . . . as it always had been. They removed the necrotic tissue, they bathed and dressed him, a few days in the hospital and he would go home with Eloise.

This time it was different. . . . They operated, they cleaned his wounds, they seemed determined. . . . He didn't get out of bed, but the infection went on advancing. . . .

It was last month when Dr. Moore told him. . . . Without hesitating, he told him, "Look, Frank, we're going to have to amputate. . . ."

He had hurt himself a little, the day before the operation, cutting his toenails . . . and it still hurt him right now! . . . as if he still had the toe! . . .

It was over now . . . it was all over. Now, he hopes . . . the problems are done with. They cut off the left one . . . but saved his life!

It all started with the swollen knee . . . (or with the arteriography?). . . . One day, he urinated blood and the doctor told Eloise to call a urologist . . . but in the arteriography it seems there was a problem. Dr. Insom said that he probably had undulating arteries in the groin . . . he fainted . . . and it seems he had an awful time . . . but Eloise didn't want them to hospitalize him. . . .

The swelling in the knee started right away . . . but they drained the pus and sent him home. . . .

He felt the first sharp pains in Smallville. . . . They went to the flower festival there. . . . Eloise loves plants! It was still hard for him to walk, but it was a nice day . . . on a bench, a couple was kissing. . . .

'85! . . . what a shitty year. . . . Florence had died of a cerebral hemorrhage . . . of his eight brothers, only one was left! . . . before his sixty-sixth birthday! . . .

Forty years! . . . always a judge's secretary in the Justice Department . . . after all, what was it all worth . . . what use was it to be responsible? . . . it was all parsimony . . . like in the morning in the hospital . . . but what would he gain by getting angry . . . he had to keep calm. . . .

After he had been forced to retire from his job, he rested for five months . . . and then a secretary again . . . doing the accounting for the Company. Always the same. . . . Eloise always said . . . that the responsibility was theirs . . . the Executive Committee's . . . why should he worry . . . he was only the secretary . . . but he suffered anyway! . . .

Forty years of marriage! . . . always praying to God for the well-being of his family . . . of the wife he had. . . . No children . . . but always companions. . . .

Eloise is good . . . a bit strong. She can withstand it better. . . .

She always risked everything for him, she always defended him . . . and now this! just when he was about to stop working . . . when he thought they could enjoy themselves a bit. . . .

He was still working when he urinated blood. . . . Carmen died very soon after and only Peter, his younger brother, was left. . . . In '85! . . . his father-in-law died too . . . he loved him so much . . . and he left him so alone. . . .

When they married, he had given them the house where they still lived. . . . Well, so to speak . . . he hasn't seen his house for a year and a half. Sometimes, in the morning, in the hospital, he feels very sad. . . .

Why are his memories fading away? . . . The house's nooks and crannies . . . sometimes, he can't quite remember what they were like. . . . And he tries to think again . . . and . . . and the club! . . . where they used to play cards, that closed down in '85. . . .

What a shitty year! he didn't go to bed with Eloise anymore after that . . . the business with his knee. . . . And he was so tired, too. . . . For a long time they'd hardly been doing it. . . . Eloise almost never had an orgasm . . . but it had always been that way, right from the beginning . . . although he'd always made an effort. . . .

Why hadn't he ever talked to anybody about it? . . . because it was always his biggest worry. . . . Why did he think so much while he was in the hospital . . . why did he look back on everything. . . .

Eloise had had some treatments, but they never found out why she didn't get pregnant. Not like Mamma . . . who had had nine children. . . . She was Armenian . . . like Pappa . . . they came over together . . . in '95 . . . and got married here.

Dad had a general store in Prescott. He was always poor, he never got ahead . . . he died at 64 of cancer. . . . She was stronger . . . she organized everything in the family . . . she lived to 77, when her heart failed. . . . She always took care of the house. . . .

Frank's history clearly shows how his life is crumbling. It all happened "at the same time," when he was about to stop working . . . when he thought that they could enjoy themselves a bit. . . . In '85: the hematuria, the arteriography, the swelling in the knee and the osteomyelitis. That same year, Florence, Carmen and then his father-in-law died, and the club where he played cards also closed down that year. From then on, he's been living "in the midst of the rubble," for a year and a half now. The deterioration is constant, the infection advances, the operations follow one after the other, finally the amputation, and then the anger, the sadness, and the unexpected condemnation of looking back on everything.

He doesn't feel secure; his father-in-law, who protected him, has died. Eloise is the one who takes care of him, but perhaps she made a mistake the first time when she didn't want him to be hospitalized, when they removed the pus from his knee and sent him home.

His habits and customs, nearly unmodified, covered up a feeling of unbearable insecurity. A certain rigidity of character defended him from instability. He was always a secretary, he always lived in the same place. The word "always" described his way of making an artificial stability for himself.

Frank shouldn't be like his father, who was always poor, who never got ahead, who was weaker than his mother. He resisted being like him and, perhaps because of that, without realizing it, he was never able to learn from those who, in some way, represented Dad. He could only be docile and chronically follow their example, obey.

As responsible as he felt, he couldn't be the boss, he was only the secretary. And now that the death of his father-in-law, who bought him a house and established his home, left the place of head of the family open, Frank wasn't able to establish himself.

The feeling of falling to pieces, however, is not conscious. When he was hospitalized, he thought that it would be for only a few days . . . also, if he says that '85 was a shitty year, it's because he thinks that better ones are ahead and that after the amputation his problems will be over. The day before the operation, he even cut the toenails of the foot they were going to amputate!

Leaving aside the infection (osteitis and myelitis), which we do not interpret at this time, we think that Frank's osteomyelitis, involving a focus of necrotic bone surrounded by an area of bone resorption and decalcification, resulted from the hypercathexis of the osteoclast process of bone resorption, a process which, when within normal limits, is part of the innervation key of the feeling of falling to pieces. We also believe that the hypercathexis occurred because this feeling, removed from consciousness, had undergone a pathosomatic deformation.

Instead of interpreting the different meanings that Frank's "organic" structures and functions communicate to us through the different illnesses that are part of his deterioration, we are interested in understanding what it is in his life that has broken down.

He felt the first sharp pains in Smallville, with Eloise, it was a nice day . . . on a bench a couple was kissing. . . . Eloise almost never had an orgasm . . . it had always been like that . . . although he'd always made an effort. . . . In this way, Frank tells us of his genital frustration, the frustration of desires that, when he is about to retire, when the time has arrived, now or never, for them to enjoy themselves a bit, threaten to break through the "moral" dams with which he has always held them back, and break up the relationships that, from the "outside," might give him the feeling of security that he lacks.

These dams, part of his normative system, which he tells us about when he refers to his responsibility in the Justice Department and in his accounting job in the Company, have already cracked. Forty years! . . . always a secretary . . . Forty years married! . . . always praying to God for his family's well-being . . . with no children . . . without satisfactory sex. After all, what was it worth . . . if everything was parsimony . . . like in the morning, in the hospital! . . .

He had to keep calm, he couldn't admit now, nearly at the end of his life, that the ethics that had always supported him and his wife, a bit strong . . . who withstands it better . . . the daughter of his father-in-law, by whom he had felt protected, could both be rigid mistakes of his own.

Thus, keeping cool and with no hopes of seeing his home again, which he cannot even remember anymore, he and his bones keep falling to pieces. Unable to admit it, he is downheartedly and resignedly on his way to death.

7

VASCULAR HEADACHES AND CEREBROVASCULAR ACCIDENTS

L. A. Chiozza, S. Aizenberg, D. Busch

I. Introduction

The most frequent of all the diverse affections of the brain are circulatory disorders, which account for 75%. They cause about 10% of all deaths worldwide and rank as the third most frequent cause of death, after cardiac disease and malignant tumors. Furthermore, ischemic hemiplegia accounts for one of the largest subgroups of patients with neuromuscular disorders (Farreras Valenti & Rozman, 1982; Stein, 1987).

    Clinical medicine has established that vascular headaches affect more patients than any other type of headache. Of this dominant group, migraine, or hemicranial headache, is the most typical. One of the clinical forms of headache, migraine with complications map present symptoms and signs of permanent and irreversible cerebral alterations ("hemiplegic migraine"), similar to those of ischemic hemiplegia. Also, among the prodromal phenomena of classical migraine, auras consisting of hemilateral paresthesias or pareses and aphasic disorders are frequently observed. On the other hand, in transient ischemic attacks, reversible neurological symptoms very similar to those of migraine can also be observed. If we consider that there are intermediate states between the lesions of migraine and those of ischemic hemiplegia, we can establish a conceptual link from the clinical and physiopathological point of view between vascular headaches and cerebral infarcts or strokes, a transition that could be considered analogous to the "continuous series" of the ischemic cardiac disorders in clinical medicine (Caino & Sanchez, 1978) and psychoanalysis (Chiozza et al., 1982).

Adding to these considerations and taking into account that the modifications in blood flow are a factor in the focal lesions of the central nervous system (Arana Iñiguez & Rebollo, 1954), we think that it is possible to establish the existence of a "family" of cerebrovascular disorders that would include vascular headaches in general as well as arteriosclerosis and cerebral infarct.

II. BRAIN FUNCTIONING

Over the course of zoological evolution, the nervous system appeared for the first time in coelenterates. It was an important advance from the previous humoral physiology, which, however, it has not replaced (Weisz, 1971). The general excitability of protoplasm furnished the starting point for the evolution of the nervous system, which links the sensory functions of organisms with their motor and vegetative functions (Freud, 1950a). Perception and movement are integrated in an inseparable functional unit (Weizsaecker, 1950b). The specific internal medium (which differs from the internal medium of the rest of the organism) and the secretion of neurohormones and neurotransmitters[1] represent the specific humoral aspects of the central nervous system (Vincent, 1986).

Freud (1950a) thought that the "system of neurons" was constituted by various subsystems. At present, the brain is thought to be not just one organ but the combination of many, each with its particular structure and its own way of reacting (Cobb, 1954; Taylor, 1979). This set of organs acts like a "biological computer," with three peculiar forms of functioning that correlate with the "three brains" described by Mac Lean (1984): the "reptile" brain, related to self-preservation; the "rodent" brain, related to emotional processes; and the "mammal brain," involved in thought processes. It is asserted that these three forms of functioning must be properly interrelated. According to Mac Lean, because of the "exponential" growth of the neocortex ("the cold brain") in human beings, the connection between the neocortex, the archeoencephalon, and the paleoencephalon ("the hot brain") has become

---

[1]In phylogenesis, excitability and the motor function are distinguished only by functional cell differentiation. In this way, the nervous system can begin to store information and to defer motor discharge (Freud, 1950a; Lorenz, 1976). The functional complex organization is structured upon the simplest elements, the reflex acts, which allows us to identify, as in any "control device," five essential components: receptor, sensory channel, modulator, motor channel, and effector (Weisz, 1971). The stimuli generated by needs (instincts) involve an "internal sensory system" with its own receptors (Freud, 1950a). The activity of the modulators is based on the modification of the impulses, the selection of the proper output channel, and the interruption, deviation, or commutation of a certain transmission chain (Weisz, 1971).

insufficient or inadequate, a characteristic that he calls "schizophysi-ology" (Mac Lean, 1984).[2]

We must stress the importance of the volume and stability of the blood flow for cerebral functioning. Although it accounts for only 2% of total body weight, the brain receives and consumes around 20% of the cardiac output and of the inspired oxygen. The adult brain, with a normal weight of 1,400 gm, thus receives approximately 1 liter of every 4 liters pumped by the heart. This quantity is more than half of that re-ceived by the liver, which is larger and heavier and whose metabolism is also important. The autonomic nervous system regulates the caliber of the cerebral arteries through localized ganglia and diffuse distribu-tion points (Cobb, 1954; Arana Iñiguez & Rebollo, 1954; Solomon et al., 1988). However, unlike muscles, the heart, and other organs, the char-acteristics of the brain prevent it from significantly increasing blood flow when metabolic needs intensify. According to neurophysiologists, when cellular activity is highly increased, if the demand of oxygen is propor-tionately greater than the supply, hypoxia phenomena take place even if there is vasodilation of the cerebral arteries (Cobb, 1954, p. 137; Arana Iñiguez & Rebollo, 1954). The circulation of the cerebrum fluctuates less and requires more stability than that of any other organ.[3] Thus, it is more sensitive than the rest of the organs to alterations in the general circulation conditions.

III. HEADACHES FROM THE CLINICAL VIEWPOINT

A. ETIOLOGY AND PATHOGENESIS

Headaches are a group of disorders involving different etiologies and pathogenetic mechanisms which affect more than 40% of the popula-tion (Ryan & Ryan, 1980; Bartleson, 1983) and are extremely frequent in occurrence. The most widely acknowledged etiologic factors in the headache syndrome are the following:

---

[2]Investigations initiated in the 1960's led to the discovery that the two cerebral hemispheres exercise different functions, and it was found that in right-handed subjects the left hemisphere is "dominant." Although right-handed people predominate, there are different degrees or combina-tions of the functions of either cerebral hemisphere. In left-handed men there is not such a clear predominance of the right hemisphere; something similar has been observed in women (Sperry, 1962; Kimura, 1973; Blakeslee, 1980). The "dominant" hemisphere is linked to the operation of logical or rational thought, analytic capacity, critical functions, and verbal language; it is usually compared to a digital computer. The "nondominant" hemisphere, considered "mute" since its func-tions are not linked to verbal language, draws away from consciousness, specializing in the es-tablishment of classes and importances, in contextual and configurational comprehension, in intuition, in the development of artistic abilities, and in nonverbal language. It is usually com-pared to an analog computer (Kimura, 1973; Watzlawick, 1977; Taylor, 1979).

[3]Ten seconds without cerebral blood flow cause neurological manifestations, including slow-ing of the EEG. After only 3 to 5 minutes during which oxygenated blood fails to reach the brain, ischemic necrotic lesions occur (Farreras Valenti & Rozman, 1982).

Irritation of the nerve fibers
Passive or active distension of the walls of blood vessels
Abnormal mechanical stimulation
Abnormal chemical stimulation
Abnormal substances
Hypoxia

As noted above, the largest percentage of headache syndromes are in the group of vascular headaches, caused by vasomotor disorders. Both headache and migraine belong to this group. Migraine is usually distinguished from the other vascular headaches, especially because it is unilateral. Migraine is also the most typical example of this group and perhaps this is the reason that most investigation concentrates on it, as we shall see when we take up its pathophysiology. We have found no reference to, or explanation of, its unilaterality in the clinical and/or neurological literature.

Pharmacological treatment of headaches is still empirical (Ryan & Ryan, 1980). Symptomatic medication is commonly used; the choice of preventive medication depends on the pathophysiological theories deemed pertinent.

B. Clinical Forms of Migraine

Migraine is a recurrent unilateral disorder in the frontotemporal or temporo-orbital zones which usually begins in puberty and decreases in frequency notably after age 50. It is somewhat more frequent in women, and 50% of patients have a family history of it, particularly in the maternal line (Farreras Valenti & Rozman, 1982).

Depending on the nature and severity of the associated symptoms, the clinical forms are the following.

Classical migraine, or hemicranial headache. Since it is considered the prototype of the "vascular headache," we shall describe its clinical symptoms in more detail than the other types. There are four phases:

1. Premonitory phase: these are fairly indefinite phenomena, including particularly dyspepsia, lack of appetite, and nervousness.
2. Prodromal phase or migraine aura. Also called "neurological phase," it is nearly constant and can take on different forms:
   a. Visual: the most frequent. Characterized by the so-called "intensification spectrum" lasting around 20 minutes. It begins as a scintillating, central, or paracentral blind spot or scotoma with serrated edges; it gradually grows outwards and at the same time becomes blindingly intense.

     b. Sensitive: manifest as hemilateral paresthesia or a tingling sensation.
     c. Sensory (nonvisual): especially cochlear, vestibular, or olfactory disorders.
     d. Aphasic disorders.
     e. Hemilateral pareses
3. Pain phase. Also called the migraine per se, it is a pulsating, intense headache that lasts for several hours, associated with some psychical disorientation. The patient is bothered by light and noise and usually lies down in the dark. The headache is frequently associated with nausea and may include vomiting. The superficial temporal artery can often be seen to be swollen and throbbing.
4. Final phase. The pain subsides, gradually becoming dull, and mentation increases. Some degree of muscular contraction may persist.
5. Electroencephalic alterations can be registered in some patients; their curves are of the epileptic type to a greater or lesser extent. Arrhythmias are found, especially in the patient with scintillating scotomas, a cortical reaction commonly persisting, as in epileptics, in response to light (Ryan & Ryan, 1980).

Common migraine or headache. This is the most frequent type of headache, the one that most people suffer from occasionally. There is no aura; the pain is only sometimes throbbing and its localizations vary; there are generally no gastrointestinal symptoms.

Migraine with complications. This form is characterized by serious neurological phenomena, ranging from cerebral edema to irreversible ischemic lesions (stroke or infarct) that may leave persistent neurological sequelae. Some investigators (Rascol et al., 1979; Bartleson, 1983) call this clinical form "hemiplegic migraine" and report that it is usually observed in patients who are younger than those who experience cerebrovascular accidents, and that atheromas in the cerebral arteries are therefore unlikely. The infarct is attributed either to the ischemic deficiency or to thrombus caused by increased platelet aggregation.

C. PATHOPHYSIOLOGY OF MIGRAINE

Although there are exceptions (Raskin et al., 1987), neurophysiologists generally agree that the encephalic mass has no receptors for pain stimuli and suggest that the only intracranial structures that do are blood vessels and some sectors of the meninges (Guyton, 1971; Farreras Valenti & Rozman, 1982). Therefore, it is usually said that the brain is "insensitive to pain."

Today, neurophysiologists agree that the vascular spasm is a multifactorial event, caused by neurogenic, biochemical, or mechanical factors that intervene alone or in combination. They have also established that persons who suffer from migraine have a labile and hyperreactive cerebrovascular system and elevated sympathetic tone that determine a persistent degree of vasoconstriction, even during migraine-free periods (Cobb, 1954; Arana Iñiguez & Rebollo, 1954; Gelmers, 1985; Solomon et al., 1988). They also accept the existence of transient stenoses provoked by neurogenic or biochemical mechanisms, demonstrable by angiography, as well as long-lasting stenoses caused by lesions of arteries that develop as a result of spasms and involve structural damage to the endothelium that can trigger a thrombosis (Solomon et al., 1988).

The different theories about the migraine attack attempt to explain the pain mechanisms. Some authors think that although the vascular spasm can be demonstrated in many patients, it is not always associated with pain, since the pain can occur without the concomitant arterial narrowing (Solomon et al., 1988). Below, we describe the most widely known hypotheses.

Humoral model. Wolff suggested that humoral control of the blood vessels was defective during the attack and identified a series of substances that accumulate around the dilated arteries and sensitize them so that otherwise innocuous stimuli cause pain: amines (serotonin, catecholamines, histamine), polypeptides (bradykinin, angiotensin), prostaglandins, and adenosine monophosphate (Wolff, 1972). Some authors (Raskin et al., 1987; Raskin, 1988) consider the vascular spasm an epiphenomenon of alterations occurring in the intracerebral pain-modulating systems that operate through serotonergic neurotransmission; these alterations are caused by a hereditary instability of these systems. Other neurophysiologists (Lechin & Van der Dijs, 1980) believe that there is an imbalance in the autonomic nervous system: in headache patients of the depressive type, the serotonergic system predominates, whereas in hypomanics the catecholaminergic system is dominant.

Hypoxia model. Although the clinical sequence suggested by Wolff is generally accepted, recent investigations have led to a theory we find more convincing: in contrast to earlier theory, a more detailed study of the characteristics of cerebral blood flow indicates that it is oligemia rather than hyperemia which produces the painful phase of migraine. This oligemia generally begins in the occipitoparietal region, gradually spreading to the entire hemisphere. It has been shown that the development of the oligemia does not correlate with the anatomical distribution of the territory of an artery or of one of its branches, as formerly believed, but that it spreads throughout the cortex of that hemisphere, which suggests a cortical, functional, and generalized alteration (Olesen et al., 1981). The migraine attack is frequently preceded by a state of neuronal excitation that is thought to lead to a focal increase in metabolism, thus raising the local oxygen requirements of the tissues (Gelmers, 1985).

The spread of the visual aura of migraine (the intensification spectrum) during the "neurological phase" is very similar to the phenomenon of diffuse cortical depression described by Leao (1944): both consist in the progression of an inhibitory wave preceded by a phase of brief neuronal activation. This coincidence suggests that the vascular changes are secondary to a primary functional disorder of the cerebral parenchyma (Gelmers, 1985).

According to this model, cortical depression is the result of previous cerebral hypoxia. The model asserts that the pre-existing rise in sympathetic tone impedes the vasodilation that is necessary to respond to metabolic requirements increased by neuronal excitation. A maladjustment between demand and supply results, thus aggravating the previous hypoxia (Gelmers, 1985). The metabolic alteration causes the discharge of substances capable of producing pain (Guyton, 1971). Investigators today agree in interpreting the arterial vasodilation of the "throbbing phase" as a subsequent compensatory reaction (Ryan & Ryan, 1980).

In summary, the fact of an intimate and reciprocal interaction between neuronal activity and cerebral blood flow leads the various authors to think that the primary element in migraine is a functional (metabolic) alteration of the cerebral parenchyma (Cobb, 1954; Arana Iñiguez & Rebollo, 1954; Gelmers, 1985; Raskin, 1988a, 1989). This means that through the liberation of pain-causing substances and vegetative irritation, which increases vascular hyperactivity, the secondary manifestations of this functional neuronal alteration are the pain phenomena and the throbbing vasodilation.

IV. CEREBROVASCULAR ACCIDENTS
FROM THE CLINICAL STANDPOINT

Of all the encephalic (brain, cerebellum, pons, medulla oblongata) circulatory disorders, cerebrovascular accidents are the most frequent (Farreras Valenti & Rozman, 1982; Stein, 1987). They are caused by alterations in cerebral circulation that occur predominantly in middle age and later years. They usually begin suddenly or acutely and evolve in a few seconds, minutes, or hours into neurological disorders, sometimes reversible, of varying severity. In some countries the term "ictus" is used only for attacks caused by a cerebral infarct or stroke that does not produce a state of coma, and the term "apoplegia" is reserved for attacks characterized by coma (Farreras Valenti & Rozman, 1982; Stein, 1987).

A. ETIOLOGY AND PATHOPHYSIOLOGY
OF CEREBROVASCULAR ACCIDENTS

The most widely accepted etiologic and pathophysiologic classification differentiates two large groups, hemorrhagic and ischemic (Stein, 1987). According to statistical reports, 10–15% of all cerebrovascular accidents are hemorrhagic. They are categorized as:

1. Spontaneous intracerebral hemorrhage
   Due to hypertension
   Due to amyloid angiopathy
   Spontaneous intracerebral hemorrhage occur most frequently in the internal capsule and, in most cases, as a result of hypertension.
2. Rupture of an aneurysm
   Congenital
   Acquired, generally mycotic
   A hemorrhage which is usually ventricular or subarachnoid (applies to both).
3. Rupture of an arteriovenous malformation
4. Trauma (*produces an extradural or subdural hematoma*)
5. Bleeding cerebral tumors
6. Systemic hemorrhagic disorders
7. Hemorrhagic cerebral infarcts

Ischemic accidents. Statistical reports indicate 85–90% of all cerebrovascular accidents (CVA) are ischemic accidents, most of which produce cerebral infarcts or strokes. It is believed that cerebral ischemia is always cardiogenic (embolic) or atherogenic (thrombotic or embolic), and it is estimated that within this group, only 10% of the total are ischemias caused by emboli originating in the heart. The largest proportion of CVAs (70–80%) results from ischemia due to atherosclerosis.

The most frequent causes of occlusive cerebral disease are thought to be the following (Stein, 1987):

Arterial
 1. Atherosclerosis
 2. Vasculitis
   a. Collagen vascular diseases
   b. Meningitis: tuberculosis, mycoses, syphilis, bacteria, herpes
 3. Vascular spasm
   a. Subarachnoid hemorrhage
   b. Migraine (mechanisms causing)
   c. Malignant hypertension

    4. Hematologic disorders
      a. Polycythemia
      b. Thrombocytopenic purpura
      c. Disseminated intravascular coagulation
      d. Dysproteinemias. Anemias
    5. Arterial dissection

Venous
    1. Paracranial infection
    2. Dehydration
    3. Systemic carcinoma
    4. Hematologic disorders
    5. Postpartum and postoperative states

Of all CVAs, 10–15% are caused by hemorrhages. Since they are not as frequent or typical, we will exclude them from our investigation, whose objective is to establish the connection between vascular headaches and ischemic CVA. However, we must discuss other ischemic disorders, the transient or reversible cases, since we believe they may provide this connection.[4] Many authors attach great importance to the previous existence of arterial hypertension (malignant or not) in relation to the CVA and maintain that atherosclerosis of the cerebral arteries is generally associated with it. Statistical data (Farreras Valenti & Rozman, 1982) show that hypertensive patients have cerebrovascular accidents five times more frequently than those who are normotensive. For these authors, arterial hypertension is the foremost risk factor in the production of ictus in general. They further believe that episodes of severe and sustained arterial hypotension can also produce cerebral infarct.

B. PATHOPHYSIOLOGY OF ISCHEMIA AND CEREBRAL INFARCT

Brain functioning depends on the stability and volume of blood flow. The longer the period without perfusion, the more irreversible the alteration of cells and function. If circulation is immediately re-established, cerebral function is completely recovered. When the ischemia lasts for a few minutes, a neuronal lesion results, and although circulation recommences, cerebral functioning takes hours to return or may not return at all. This is caused by the failure of the affected capillaries to recanalize, which impedes the re-establishment of flow. Prolonged ischemia leads to necrosis of the affected cerebral tissue (infarct), followed by cerebral edema in 24–48 hours (Stein, 1987).

---

[4]It is significant that in the above etiological classification vascular spasms have been included and within them, migraine.

Atherosclerosis of the cerebral arteries is usually most extensive at the forks of the internal carotid and its intracranial branches. In general, the severity of the atherosclerotic process determines the probability of an ischemic attack. However, there is no direct or linear correlation, since other factors are operative, including the integrity of the collateral circulation, the state of the cardiovascular system, and possibly hematological factors. Some patients with massive infarcts have minimal atherosclerosis, whereas others have one or more main arteries occluded and are totally free of ischemic symptoms (Stein, 1987).

The atherosclerotic plaques cause arterial stenosis and, therefore, obstruction of cerebral blood flow; if for any reason it falls below the critical level a transient or permanent ischemic accident occurs. The ulceration of plaques of atheroma can lead either to an embolism caused by the breaking away of necrotic material or to the formation of a thrombus due to agglutination of platelets and coagulation of fibrin. Either of these processes is capable of obstructing a blood vessel (Stein, 1987).

The contribution of vascular spasm to ischemia and infarction is subject to discussion. Some authors (Stein, 1987; Solomon et al., 1988) suggest that vascular spasm may always be involved in the genesis of the ischemia or infarction, either as a triggering factor or as a factor associated with other mechanisms. Analogous questions have been raised regarding the role of vessel spasm in the etiology of myocardial infarction (Chiozza et al., 1982); it is to be hoped that future investigations will clear up this point.

The pathophysiology of the edema associated with cerebral ischemia is so characteristic that many authors call it "ischemic edema" (Stein, 1987). This edema is due to a cytological factor, produced by a defect in the sodium pump at the level of the cell membranes, which produces an accumulation of intracellular water. This toxin develops in the first few minutes following the accident and produces tumefaction of the neuroglia, the neurons, and the endothelial cells of the capillaries. Later, the so-called vasogenic factor, predominating in the white substance, is brought on by an increase in capillary permeability that destroys the blood–brain barrier and allows the passage of proteins from the blood to the extravascular space. When circulation is rapidly re-established, the cytotoxic edema leaves no sequelae. If not, this edema causes the phenomena of non-recanalization, supporting the maintenance of the ischemia and consequent necrosis. When the edema advances to the vasogenic phase and remains there, the extent of the infarct usually increases progressively (Stein, 1987).

C. Clinical Forms of Ischemic CVA

The symptoms of the cerebrovascular accident depend on the extent, localization, and temporal evolution of the ischemia (Stein, 1987).

Depending on their extent, infarcts are classified as focal or massive. The occlusive or obstructive vascular lesion may be in the carotid territory or its branches, the most frequent sites being the internal capsule or in the vertebrobasilar territory or its branches.

The effects of the ischemic attack also depend on its temporal evolution and may take one of the following forms.

Transient ischemic attack (TIA). These last from 5 to 30 minutes and resolve completely within 24 hours, leaving no sequelae. The usual symptoms are:

1. Motor: hemipareses or contralateral monoparesis. These are the most frequent.
2. Sensory: contralateral paresthesia
3. Ocular: ipsilateral amaurosis. Infrequent, associated with pain in the eye and the forehead.
4. Dysarthria or dysphasia: when the ischemia occurs in the dominant hemisphere

Reversible ischemic neurological deficiency. Signs and symptoms of a TIA but lasting longer than 24 hours with complete clinical recovery and no sequelae.

Progressive or evolving attack. Symptoms are aggravated and finally develop into a full attack.

Full attack. With an established infarct. The neurological symptoms depend on the arterial territory affected, the degree of occlusion, and the importance of the occluded vessel.

In this study, we focus on the most frequent and typical ictus, meaning those whose complete clinical manifestation is hemiplegia. Since these CVAs result from insufficiencies in the carotid artery or its branches, they depend on alterations occurring particularly in the internal capsule, an area irrigated by the medium cerebral artery, which is a branch of the internal carotid. We will not discuss focal accidents or those involving insufficiencies in the vertebrobasilar territory.

The middle cerebral artery supplies large sectors of the frontal, temporal, and parietal lobes. Since the "favorite" and most frequent and typical site of the lesion is the proximal part of the artery, the most affected area is the internal capsule, an area of white substance through which most of the motor (ventral) and sensory (dorsal) fibers run, leading to or away from these lobes (Jimenez Diaz, 1936; Fracassi, 1945). Consequently, the following symptoms are produced:

1. Motor: generally severe contralateral hemiplegia.
2. Sensory: contralateral hemianesthesia.
3. Ocular: homonymous or ipsilateral hemianopsia, frequently accompanied by deviation of the head and paresis of the internal facial nerve.
4. Cerebral edema: extensive, manifested clinically by alteration of the level of consciousness, including even deep coma.
5. Aphasia: occurs when the dominant hemisphere is affected; apraxia or anosognosia results when the nondominant hemisphere is affected.

By 24–48 hours after the ictus has begun, certain muscle groups are usually affected with flaccid paralysis, and the reflexes are altered.[5] A few days later, the paralysis becomes spastic, forming the typical hemiplegic condition: the upper extremity is usually more seriously affected than the lower. The arm is adducent, the forearm rigid, flexed, and pronate, with the fingers subjected to contractures and flexed. The fine movements of the hands and fingers are difficult to recover and the hand remains in forced and spastic pronation so that the patient must learn to do everything with the other hand. The affected leg usually becomes useful again for walking but in a "peg-legged" manner. Because of this, the hemiplegic is described as having "the reaper's gait" (Farreras Valenti & Rozman, 1982).

V. THE PSYCHOANALYTIC VIEW OF VASCULAR
HEADACHES AND CEREBROVASCULAR ACCIDENTS

A. PSYCHOANALYTIC BASES

Freud suffered from migraines (Jones, 1953–1957) and referred to the disorder several times. In some letters (Freud, 1950a, Letter 59, April 6, 1897 [S.E. 1:244], and Draft I, undated [S.E. 1:213]) and papers (1895b), he signalled its relation to disturbed sexual discharge; he also interpreted it as a symbolic displacement of a fantasy of rape (Freud, 1950a, Letter 102, Jan. 16, 1899 [S.E. 1:277]). When he referred to the forgetting of names (1901b), he stated that this phenomenon sometimes preceded his own migraines, connecting it with personal circumstances that provoked intense and painful affects. After Freud, several authors have taken up such research. Fenichel (1957) indicated that headaches often symbolize

---

[5]Hemiplegic paralysis follows the so-called Wernikke Mann Law of prediction: in the upper limb the opposition of the thumb and the supination of the hand paralyze early; the same happens to the extensor muscles and the muscles participating in supination of the forearm. In the lower extremity, the flexor muscles are much more affected than the extensors. This selective distribution of the paralysis depends not only on the extent to which each muscle is affected but also on the modification of the reflexes of distension-shortening typical of each muscle (Jimenez Diaz, 1936).

fantasies of pregnancy. He also found that when an unconscious hostile tendency is meant to destroy an object's intelligence, guilt feelings orient this tendency against the subject's own head. Garma (1970) also maintained that genitality disorders and repressed hostility are basic factors that trigger the attacks. Brenner et al. (1949) expressed similar ideas. Garma (1958, 1969) and other authors (Cárcamo, 1944) observed a higher frequency of migraine in patients suffering from obsessional neurosis, characterized by the "blockage" of emotions by processes of rationalization. Garma (unpublished report[6]) connected the ocular pain of migraine to the blinding light involved in the birth trauma. Pichon-Rivière (1943) related migraine to epilepsy and ambivalent feelings.

In regard to hemiplegia, the only reference in the psychoanalytic literature is in Freud's book on President Wilson (Freud & Bullit, 1966). Wilson suffered from intense headaches and had several "collapses" at important moments in his life, breakdowns Freud considered to be antecedents of the left-sided hemiplegia he suffered in 1919.[7]

Although these investigations are valuable forerunners, they fall short of providing complete understanding of the disorder—in particular, of the elements determining the choice of the affected organ and its unconscious meaning.

B. Specific Unconscious Meanings

The natural continuation of a line of thought initiated by Freud has led us to postulate that, as compared to neurosis and psychosis, somatic illness involves a different type of defense, i.e., way of making the terms of a conflict unconscious, in which the conflict is expressed in disguise by the physical symptoms (Chiozza, 1963, 1970a, 1971a).

Somatic illness can be interpreted as a form of language since it is able to convey meaning.

In stating the second basic hypothesis of psychoanalysis, Freud (1940a) started from the fact that conscious psychical sequences are incomplete, or broken. If the psychical is held to be identical with consciousness, physical or somatic processes concomitant with what is psychical would have to be postulated to account for the broken conscious psychical sequences. Freud, however, asserted psychoanalysis's

[6]Garma, A., "Fundamental aspects of resistances in the final stages of psychoanalytical treatment," presented at the Argentine Psychoanalytical Association, Buenos Aires, 1972.

[7]Freud and Bullit (1966) described two "collapses" in the life of Wilson, one in 1906 and the other in 1908. Both involved great nervousness, upset stomach, and bilious headache. In the episode in 1906, he suffered the rupture of an artery of the retina in the left eye, which left him partially blind, but he also had pain in his left shoulder and leg, which were attributed to a neuritis. Both episodes, like the one that provoked the hemiplegia in 1919, occurred during intense political campaigns, and Freud interpreted the breakdowns as expressions of his intense unconscious masculine–feminine conflicts in relation to the paternal figure, which returned because of the repetition compulsion.

second basic hypothesis, that is, that there exists a psychic unconscious. He implied that it is in the domain of the unconscious that the sequences required to complete and explain the broken conscious sequences are to be found.

In view of Freud's ideas, we are of the opinion that in our conscious knowledge of ourselves and of others, we define as "somatic" the unconscious processes that reach consciousness only as a sensorial perception while their meaning remains unconscious. (When the meaning of crying remains unconscious, lachrymal secretion is categorized by the person as epiphora, since he/she perceives it only as a physical phenomenon) (Chiozza, 1981a).

The main points of the theory to which we subscribe are the following:

1. It is possible to find an unconscious meaning inherent in any somatic form, function, or process, either normal or pathological. The existence of that meaning shows that the body is capable of symbolic function (Chiozza, 1963).
2. Every physical process therefore correlates to an unconscious fantasy that is specific to that process or inherent in it (Chiozza, 1963). We view somatic illnesses as particular combinations or "mosaics" of different specific fantasies (Chiozza, 1970a).
3. The somatic processes that consciousness interprets as phenomena stripped of affective meaning are discharge processes produced by an affective innervation key, deformed by repression, a key that configures the unconscious meaning of the somatic process (Chiozza, 1976a, 1978a).

This is our theoretical basis when we refer to the specific unconscious meanings of headaches and hemiplegias.

C. THE BRAIN AND THE HEAD

In an earlier work (Chiozza, 1980a), we used the cybernetic model to represent the specific "cerebral" fantasies as formal configurations of integration, equivalent to negative feedback circuits. This model, used to represent what is "cerebral" in general, enables us to understand that these formal configurations intervene both in the construction of a reflex and in the establishment of a judgment. However, since intelligence, knowledge, and memory are products of the whole of what we call "organism," they cannot be attributed to the brain alone. Knowing and memorizing are accomplished by the whole body, that is, by the person as a whole.

We must add that the investigation of the specific fantasies (Chiozza, 1970, 1970a) led us to postulate that any organ that participates to a greater extent in certain processes than other organs is assigned the representation of these processes. Thus, we say that "the hepatic" is assigned, by way of the liver, to the representation of the process of materialization (Chiozza, 1963), just as "the cardiac" is assigned—by way of the heart—to the representation of the emotions and "the cerebral" is assigned—by way of the brain—to the representation of the thought processes; we could say that one unconscious structure is the source of both the thought processes and the representations of brain and head that enter consciousness. Linguistic usage and also some scientific theories (Cobb, 1954; Azcoaga, 1983) confirm this conclusion, inasmuch as they, too, assert the brain and the head are the seat of the function of thinking, of intelligence, and also of the tempering of the affects.[8] To exemplify these points: when a person concentrates in order to think, he frequently grasps his forehead in his hands; the occurrence of an idea is usually signalled by placing the forefinger on the frontotemporal angle. The temple, however, is related to madness, as in the gesture that says, "This guy is nuts." It is also common to speak of "keeping one's head" to refer to the low degree of emotion involved in the exercise of reason.

D. THOUGHT AND ACTION

According to Freud (1900a, 1911b, 1950a), thought is "interiorized action" that operates through a "small quantity" of cathexis of the mnemic traces of performed actions. This is what psychoanalysis calls "tentative investing." The psyche progresses from "identity of perception" (Freud, 1900a) to "identity of thought"[9] by establishing complex associative connections. This requires the capacity for tolerating postponement of drive discharge, which thwarts the development of the full-quantity identity pertaining to the primary process that is at work in the perception. Judgment, which is the result of the secondary process, puts an end to the delay that thought itself implies and thus leads from thought to action.

---

[8]Three "brains" can be differentiated according to their phylogenetic age (Mac Lean, 1984): the archiencephalon or "reptile" brain regulates the function of the viscera and the reflex mechanisms and has an alarm system connected to sensory information. The paleoencephalon, or "rodent" brain, also called the "hot brain," integrates the emotions. Its link with the cerebellum, an organ that incorporates learned abilities and converts them into "automatic" habits (Taylor, 1979), enables us to admit the existence of affective, inherited, and acquired automatisms. The neoencephalon (neocortex), or "cold brain," is linked to the rational thought processes and to the execution of voluntary actions and is usually compared to digital computers. It is also thought to possess the very important function of inhibiting or tempering emotional behavior (Cobb, 1954). This is deduced from the observation of intense emotional reactions (attack of rage) produced by experimental lesions that free the archiencephalon and the paleoencephalon from the control (inhibition) exerted by the neoencephalon (Cobb, 1954).

[9]Psychoanalysis calls "perception identity" the identity established when an unfulfilled wish attributes to memory in the form of a hallucination the traits of the perception and allows the discharge corresponding to action with full cathexis. On the other hand, thought identity occurs when the thought process finds sufficient coincidence between the representation of the wish and that arising from perception.

We call appropriate actions those that manage to put an end to the needs that flow from the drive sources (Freud, 1950a). Therefore, it is implicit that they must be specific, and for this reason Freud (1950a) also called them specific actions. Apart from this, actions are appropriate when, whatever their efficacy may be, their meaning, their direction toward an aim and their purpose are comprehensible.

Any thought, however small the cathexis of the representations it uses may be, always involves a motor discharge (Freud, 1905d, 1950a). The discharge of a drive is always accomplished by the sum of a vegetative motor component and a motor component pertaining to relational life (i.e., the nonvegetative component of the nervous system). The former belongs to what we call affect and the latter to what we call action. Action is always associated with a quota of affective discharge, and the process of discharge that we call affect always occurs with a component of action (Freud, 1911b; Chiozza, 1974).

In view of these considerations we must infer that the cerebral vegetative processes, especially the vascular processes, are part of the normal "innervation key" of the thought processes.

Thought processes contribute to the configuration of the norms of actions. Once the efficacy of an appropriate action has been confirmed, it is preserved in unconscious memory. Both the process of constitution of a norm and its unconscious registration undergo a series of stages that range from the ideas and judgments involved in imprecise, hesitant, impulsive or tentative movements to those of the most elaborate and precise motor coordinations.

Therefore, thought and action are indissolubly united in the unconscious. This happens not only because the omnipotence of ideas—corresponding to primitive magical thinking operating in the unconscious psyche as a primary process—renders them equivalent (Freud, 1909a, 1912–1913), but also because the "innervation key" of the thought processes is always intimately included in the "innervation key" of the motor acts of relational life (Freud, 1905d, 1950a). This integration between action and thought is just as close as that between thought and experience.

E. Affects

Freud (1900a, 1915c) defined the affects as processes of discharge produced through vegetative "innervations" arising from the "full" cathexis of the unconscious ideas that constitute their "innervation keys" (Freud, 1900a). Like inherited and congenital hysterical attacks, affects correspond to the perpetuation in the present of phylogenetically appropriate actions (Freud, 1926d).

The affective discharge is one of the evidences of the excitation originating in the drive organization. When the discharge takes place in full quantity, this is a "primary affect" (Chiozza, 1976a) pertaining to what is called "passion."

The discharge of a primary affect can take place in the body itself or become action (Freud, 1950a). When this discharge is unpleasurable (contradictory) for the rest of the ego, the need to "temper" the affects arises. The conflict generated between contradictory affects may include the constitution of a compromise formation subjacent to the constitution of symptoms (Freud, 1900a, 1905d, 1950a [Letter 102, *S.E.* 1:277]).

It is clear that the work of thought, considered synonymous with the concept of psychical working-through (Freud, 1900a, 1940a, 1950a; Laplanche & Pontalis, 1967; Aizenberg, 1975), exercises the important function of tempering the affects, thanks to the relations between thought and action on the one hand and between affect and action on the other. The link can be achieved by integrating the ideational components of the conflicting affect with the ideational components of other affects or of previous thought and judgmental processes (pre-judices), that are part of the coherent ego. Sometimes, the "innervation key" of another affect is hypercathected, so that this affect completely replaces the former one, acting as a countercathexis. Thus, in one way or another, a secondary affect arises (Chiozza, 1976a), which we call "feeling." The "naming" of the primary or secondary affects, their link with adequate word-representations, is part of the process of "tempering" the affects. In this way, an impassive verbal naming process can take place totally stripped of emotion, as in the formation of logical thought.

F. "Mottos"

In this text, we use the word "motto" (in Spanish, *lema*), drawing from its original meaning of "proposition," "subject," or "premise" (Corominas, 1961), to designate a principle of action held as the result of a previously formed judgment (pre-judice) that orients behavior in a conscious or unconscious manner.

The various mottos can be considered the respective cogitative equivalents of different affects, since affects are discharged according to phylogenetically appropriate action patterns. Since the motto is a cogitative representative of the affects, it can be used to temper them.

VI. Vascular Headaches and Cerebrovascular
Accidents as Specific Unconscious Fantasies

A. Pain

Freud (1926d) included pain as an affect. From the quantitative viewpoint, pain arises when a constant or very intense stimulus cannot be avoided by effective actions. When we studied the pain associated with angina pectoris (Chiozza et al., 1982), we said that it functions as a signal whose purpose is to protect the person from an effort symbolizing another effort experienced as excessive, which remains unconscious. One could think that a headache expresses both the effort and the displeasure deriving from the unrealized attempt to transform or to dominate an affective incongruency through rationalization.

Language constantly refers to the facts we are describing. Someone worried about a serious conflict says that "it is giving him a headache." Freud (1895b) tells of a patient, Cäcilie M., for whom the headache was resolved as if it were a thought pain. "It's gotten into my head," she would say, and also, "The pain loosened up [*lösen*] when the respective problem was resolved [*lösen*]." In the headaches that occur as throbbing pain (as in the "pulsating phase" of the migraine attack), we see the most typical representation of its unconscious meaning, since in those cases the head "throbs" as if it were a heart. The common expression in Spanish, "My blood went to my head," certainly owes its origin to the—formerly conscious—perception of the fantasies involved in the headache.

B. THE COMMON HEADACHE

As noted, the need to temper the affects arises when conflict is generated by contradictory emotions. The motto, the thought representative of an affect, can be used for tempering the affects; when this is successful, the emotions are discharged through moderated or adequate words and actions. However, if the affective conflict continues, the subject is faced with a "dilemma." The dilemma involves the coexistence of two (*di-*) conflicting mottos (Real Academia Española, 1950; Corominas, 1961) and therefore represents and thus expresses the persistence of the conflict. Frequently when a person is faced with this type of alternative, he/she will scratch his/her head; the scratching implies the symbolic attempt to eliminate the excitation that cannot be worked out.

In these circumstances, the subject can resort to thought, trying to resolve the dilemma by transforming the affective conflict into an authentic rational problem. In fact, a problem is a "task proposed" to the intellect (Corominas, 1961). Through the work of thought, the subject examines and evaluates each of the mottos related to the opposite ones and also considers the present circumstances involved in the conflict, circumstances that determine variations in the applicability of each of the mottos. Through the capacity for tempering the affects operating with "small-quantity" cathexes, thinking finds an adequate and moderate thought representation, thus enabling resolution of the conflict.

If the subject uses the mottos involved in the problem of the dilemma as rationalizations, however, the subjacent affects these mottos represent cannot be tempered. An insoluble problem-dilemma then takes shape.

Many authors (Freud, 1909a; Garma, 1958; Bleger, 1967) indicate that rationalization and brooding are characteristic in patients with an obsessional structure. Many of these patients also suffer from migraine (Cárcamo, 1944; Garma, 1958, 1970; Ryan & Ryan, 1980).

We believe that in these circumstances, the patient expects (Chiozza, 1986b) "reason to triumph," trying to handle an affective conflict that remains unconscious as if it were a problem pertaining exclusively to rational thought and thus leaving the subject "impassive," without a trace of emotion. This reminds us of Pascal's dictum: "The heart has reasons that reason ignores."

The investigation of somatic illnesses led us to the conclusion that they involve a decomposition of the "innervation key" of the affects included in the present conflict. An example is the "ignominy-ischemia" typical of ischemic cardiac disorders (Chiozza et al., 1982). Since we consider the cerebral vascular processes to be part of the normal "innervation key" of the cogitative processes, it is safe to suggest that the vascular headache or the ischemic cerebral disorder that it involves is an equivalent manifestation, both expressive and symbolic, of a problem-dilemma that has become insoluble and whose importance remains unconscious.

In the case of vascular headaches, we propose that what is lost is the coherence of the "innervation keys," of the thoughts that constitute the dilemma, or of the problem that cogitatively represents the conflicting affects. Consequently, it is not the dilemma or problem or its importance that penetrate consciousness as such, but instead, the pain of the headache.

It can be assumed that when an affective conflict cannot be represented in a dilemma or in a problem, the subject is faced with a kind of cogitative "disconcertedness," which we describe as the feeling that something is "inconceivable." The term "to conceive," originally meaning to contain, to absorb (Corominas, 1961), is also defined as "to become pregnant," "to form an idea," and "to begin to feel a passion or affect" (Real Academia Española, 1950). The knowledge of these meanings leads us to consider "inconceivable" the word best suited to describe the process implicit in migraine.[10]

---

[10]We must explain our use of the terms "ignominy" and "inconceivable" in the description of the processes we are investigating. Because of their original etymological meaning, some words lack direct reference to the principal meaning that has been confirmed by use. An example of this is the case of envy: etymologically, it refers to visual processes (*invideo*) (Corominas, 1961): we know that it alludes to the visual component of the emotion of envy although its main use is that of a hepatic affect. We preferred to hold to the use of the term "ignominy," whose literal meaning is that of "something that has no name" (Corominas, 1961), to describe the affect or process linked to the ischemic cardiac disorders. We reserve the use of the term "inconceivable" for the migraine disorder. The meaning of this word, as discussed in the text, is the one that best suits as the name of the process involved in migraine (Real Academia Española, 1950; Corominas, 1961).

Everyday language alludes to this situation in expressions such as: "I don't know what to think" or "It doesn't enter my head." Garma (1958) stated that many migraine sufferers experience their emotional conflicts as "foreign objects" that "fill their head." Certain myths also express these unconscious meanings. (See sections IX and X below, referring, respectively, to the myth of the birth of Pallas Athena and the myth of Orestes.)

The unconscious meanings specific to the ischemic cerebral disorder whose clinical manifestation is migraine configure the "mosaic" of fantasies that form the set of its most frequent symptoms: scintillating scotoma, ocular pain, photophobia, nausea and vomiting, and hemicranial pain.

The intensity of the pain of migraine—usually greater than that of the common headache—is possibly constituted as a deformation of the "innervation key" of thought processes that have been unable to free themselves of a state of "disconcertedness," resulting in a dilemma. (We here apply a conceptualization analogous to that of the emotional "disconcertedness" of the ischemic cardiac disorders.)

Further, we believe that in migraine patients, who generally have an obsessional character structure, the expectation of resolving "affairs of the heart" through "reasoning" is greater. They manifest in this way their difficulty in using thought activity adequately in order to conceive creative solutions to their conflicts.

1. Scintillating scotoma and photophobia, the migraine "aura," seem to represent suitably by means of "visual" symbolism the traumatic shock of some ideal forms represented by the term "dazzling" (Chiozza, 1963, 1970).[11]

2. Nausea and vomiting symbolically represent a "hepatic" insufficiency or failure in the task of materializing or assimilating those ideal exigencies (Chiozza, 1963). This interpretation enables us to understand the unconscious meaning of the widespread belief that headaches or migraines are provoked by gallbladder or liver disorders, as expressed in the English name for migraine: bilious attack (Garma, 1958).

3. Hemicranial pain, which is so typical of migraine that it is one of its names, links the vascular headache—along with other hemilateral disturbances that are sometimes manifested, such as paresthesias, pareses,

---

[11]When we refer to the clinical forms of migraine and also when we review previous psychoanalytic investigations, we find a possible link with epilepsy. The "dazzling" luminous stimuli trigger "ocular" defense mechanisms tending to avoid the danger of destruction. This "ocular" defense can also occur with the emergence of traumatic memories having visual characteristics or visual scenes of an ideal or "dazzling" nature.

Both the visual aura in epilepsy and in migraine could be seen as manifestations of these "dazzling" ideal fantasies. One of the basic differences between the two disorders is that in epilepsy, the neuronal "irritation" is unable to reach a pattern of organized action and triggers a compulsive type of discharge. In migraine, however, the "impossible" discharge of the excitation involved occurs through ocular and cephalic pain.

or aphasias—with the symptoms of the cerebrovascular accidents that evolve under the clinical form of hemiplegia.

Clinical medicine is unable to explain the hemilaterality of these symptoms. Since the discovery that the two cerebral hemispheres have different functions and that the "dominant" hemisphere is generally related to logical thought and verbal language (Sperry, 1962; Kimura, 1973; Blakeslee, 1980), some investigators have tried to establish correlations between these characteristics and some psychosomatic affections, including migraine, but conclusions are contradictory (Gur & Gur, 1975; Blakeslee, 1980;).[12]

The concept of dissociation of the personality used in psychoanalysis (Freud, 1940a; Klein, 1954), together with knowledge of the symbolic meaning of the left (sinister aspects, sin, crime, or passion) and the right (justice and rectitude), enable us to interpret hemilaterality as an expression of the difficulty of reconciling the clashing mottos that constitute a dilemma or the affects these mottos represent. Ziegler (1986), only implicitly discussing laterality, agreed with this idea, since he pointed out that migraine expresses a conflict between "the civilized part" and "the wild part" of the subject.

4. The vasodilation of the final phase of the attack often involves transudation and edema, which account for the residual phenomena, sensory or motor, following the attack. If we consider that vasodilation generates a kind of circulatory stasis, we can suppose that it symbolizes the disheartening ("cardiac insufficiency") caused by the uselessness of the effort made to resolve the conflict. The edema seems to represent an "exudative fantasy" or an equivalent of tears (Chiozza et al., 1964), symbolizing inadequate working-through of a mourning process, also implicit in the meaning of the pain.[13]

C. HEMIPLEGIA

When the intensity of the affects that motivate thought activity is great, thought is acted out with a "high" action component. Thought is then slowed, because of the magnitude of the "full" (primary) cathexes swept along with it. We accept that it is mainly the brain or the encephalon that intervenes in thinking, and that the cerebral vascular processes are part of the "innervation key" of the thought processes. Since we conceive of the brain as a "center" directing the sensory-motor activity that configures

[12]Gur & Gur (1975) and Blakeslee (1980) found a clear predominance of migraine and immune disorders in left-handed patients whose right hemisphere dominates. Bakan (quoted by Ferguson, 1983) found the opposite.

[13]Among the main derivatives of the word "pain" (in Spanish, *dolor*), referring both to physical discomfort and to sorrow or grief, regret, and repentance (Real Academia Española, 1950), we find the term "mourning," the process that takes place after an important loss and also includes the meaning of "duel" (in Spanish, *duelo*) (Corominas, 1961).

actions, we must suppose that the vascular processes mentioned are also a part of the "innervation key" of actions. Therefore, we can assume that the ischemic disorders developing into a cerebral infarct or edema, transiently or permanently invalidating sensory-motor functions, are the expressive and symbolic equivalent of a dilemma or cogitative "disconcertedness" involving a considerable component of action. This dilemma or "disconcertedness" then remains unconscious, transferring the "whole" of its entire cathexis to the cerebral vascular-parenchymal process that normally is part of the "innervation key" of the actions involved and thus "transforms" them into a "somatic disorder" affecting the ventral and dorsal nerve roots that are linked to intentional or voluntary movement (pertinent to the so-called "sphere of relational life").

If the "disconcertedness" implicit in the hemiplegia is evidenced in disability or paralysis of the movements that configure a given action, it is understandable that the different motor and sensory signs belonging to the different clinical forms of this syndrome pertain to the different actions and affects involved in the conflict. For example, we consider that the hemiopsia of hemiplegia may be a transformation expressing the same process that is evidenced in the migraine aura as the scintillating scotoma.

When we imagine a person who has suffered a cerebral infarct, we visualize an "older man" who looks pathetic and "wrecked," who has great difficulty in walking, dragging his leg along and leaning on a cane. He is generally with his wife, who looks as though she feels sorry for him but is also intensely annoyed. The hemiplegic is unable to move his arm or to walk and seems to be "clumsy or dumb," sometimes even losing the ability to communicate. We believe that these symptoms cover up deep feelings of powerlessness and indignation, as well as intense desires for revenge, and express the inhibition of a cruel and violent action that might take shape as a homicide, a crime of passion. One of the crimes of passion we imagine is the one inspired by a feeling of having been deceived and betrayed.[14]

---

[14]The triggering of a hemiplegia generally leads to a sudden, unexpected attack; that is why it is called an "accident." The investigation of the unconscious fantasies expressed in accidents (Granel, 1975) reveals, on the one hand, a need to reach a state of unconsciousness and an allegation of "innocence" by way of resorting to "fatality" or "coincidence"; on the other hand, he pointed out that a humiliating violent scene is being dramatized through the accident.

Medical terms used to describe episodes of hemiplegia also reveal the attachment of the unconscious meaning of "ictus," referring to the attack's paroxysmal or abrupt nature (*Dorland's Diccionario de Ciencias Médicas*, 1983). The etymological meaning also conveys the idea of "hit," "hurt," "threat," or "damage" (De Miguel & Marqés de Morante, 1943).

Both the German *schlaq* (*Diccionario Etimológico de la Lengua alemana*, 1963) and the English "stroke" (Collins, 1987), used as lay equivalents to "cerebrovascular accident," mean "punch" and "fight." The original meaning of "migraine" also involves the idea of "fight." In Spanish *apoplejia* (apoplexy) refers to an episode of ictus that causes a coma and alludes to the state of being paralyzed, beaten up, or knocked down (Corominas, 1961). In English apoplexy means a "stroke" and also "a fit of extreme anger; rage" (*Webster's Collegiate Dictionary*, 1996).

An illustration of these ideas is found in a paragraph from a play by Eugenio Griffero (1982), entitled "Prince Charming":

GUSTAV: "John . . . Martha, my wife, cheated on me, years ago, in the summer, in our friends' house. From the garden, I heard Martha's voice saying, panting . . . No! Please, no! . . . Our host embraced her. . . . I heard her. . . . She resisted an instant, only an instant and then . . . then, I couldn't move . . . my heart stopped. . . . She cheated on me. Someone only had to insist for an instant for her to. . . . I can still hear it in my ears. . . . No! No! Please, no! That was it. . . . With Martha everything went on as usual. We're an excellent couple. . . . That's what I think, in spite of her stinginess and this (he points to the limp half of his body). Two years ago, John, this part of my body got tired of working and said good-bye. And I began to drag this half cadaver of mine around. Since then there are two of us and we know each other well, I complain about him, I scold him, I dress him. . . . This part of me doesn't pay any attention to me. It rests. I want to rest . . . and I get agitated as usual. . . . I'm afraid you'll see me, John. . . . I'm so old!"

VII. THE PAINFUL EXCLUSION OF A MOTTO

Caesar, aged, 40, has suffered from migraine nearly once a month since he was 12 years old, and the hemicranial pain is predominantly on the left side. His mother, also a migraine-sufferer and an alcoholic with a violent temper, was frivolous and led an irregular life. Depending on her mood in her drunkenness, one day was a party and the next a funeral.

His father, very melancholic and always ill, burdened him with responsibilities since he was very small. This man seemed to be just one more tenant in the boarding house his wife ran. Caesar was the victim of incredible beatings when he defended his father in the quarrels between father and mother.

When he was 18, taking his father's advice, he broke off with Marianne, although he liked her very much and had been going with her since they were 15, to marry Louise.

With Louise, he wants to realize his ambition of having a good, calm, and well-balanced family. Not until seven years after marrying were they able to have a child, their son Mario. Louise is a good, helpful wife and together they struggle and progress. Meanwhile, Caesar gets a degree in economics. One year after his graduation, Louise unexpectedly leaves him.

They divorce and Caesar works intensely with great sacrifice. During that period between ages 31 and 34, the headaches that have tortured him without respite since he was 12 years old go away.

At that time, he is assigned to an important post in a state enterprise. More than three years have passed since his divorce, and he meets Claudia, an architect 31 years old, divorced and the mother of two. The new family is formed when Claudia's children move in with them. Caesar cannot shake off the feeling that the passionate sexuality that she communicates to him is perpetuating a relationship between lovers that has not been consolidated as a legally sanctioned marriage. Migraines come back at this time with their usual frequency.

Claudia makes him feel, alternately, that he is in heaven or in hell. She is a sweet companion, devoted to family life, but the main barrier is her irrational violence that obeys no rule of logic. "This happens to me of all people," says Caesar, "I'm pure reason."

At present, he experiences anxiety crises and feels empty. His intense migraine attacks are increasingly frequent. Neither the usual analgesics nor ergotamin derivates relieve him and he must stay in bed. When the episode begins to go away, he feels an indescribable anxiety, the feeling of having a bomb in his head and the fear of going mad. He is assaulted by the fantasy of crashing through the railroad crossing barrier with the car. Although he has always won respect in his profession, he is afraid they will discover he is a fake.

In the first interview of his "pathobiography" (Chiozza, 1986), he tells of his first migraine episode. He was 12 years old when it happened. He threw himself onto his parents' bed (he slept in the same bed with them until he was 9, when his sister was born). He was wearing a blue sweater lent to him by his (female) cousin, with whom he had played at "everything," even at getting married. Then he vomited and it went away.

In the second interview (two days later), he is worried about the EEG and talks of his fear of madness. After the first interview, he had the worst migraine attack he had had in a long time. The pain wasn't in his eye but in his temple (he points to his left temple). He takes analgesics and tries to go to sleep. Then, while daydreaming, he "dreams" that under the sheets there was a blue folder (like the ones he uses for balance sheets and tax statements). The doctors seeing him during his pathobiography were there. The folder contained the contents of his life, or of his crises. The doctors threw him out. Then, awakening, as it were, he said that he wanted to narrate an episode that was very hard for him to communicate.

In this episode, he broke the rules he had obeyed since he was a child when he used to go to church. Two years ago, he met Marianne, his first girlfriend, in an office. He doesn't know whether it was a relationship he still cared about or whether he fell in love again. The relationship they started was very intense and passionate. He had never in his life experienced such strong feelings during sexual relations. He felt he was in heaven. Besides that, she was healthy, intelligent, and well-off. He felt loved and valued. He even thought of divorcing Claudia. When he had already been "dissuaded" (a lapsus linguae for "persuaded" or "decided"), Marianne suddenly dies in an accident.

His relationship with Marianne lasted only three months, but Caesar reasons that it was better that way. Perhaps destiny wanted to protect his family from a separation.

Caesar's whole history seems to be marked by two opposing "mottos" represented by the paternal and maternal imagos. His mother represented uncontrolled passion, violence, excitement, incest, chaos, destruction, oscillation between heaven and hell, the party and the funeral, but also vitality and pleasure. His father preached responsibility and sacrifice, calmness, equanimity, and order, progress and security, but also represented sadness and emptiness, depression, lack of satisfaction, complaint, illness, and hardship.

This dilemmatic conflict expresses Caesar's biographical vicissitudes. On the one hand, his relationship with Marianne, the illegality of his life with Claudia, the "incredible" beatings he received from his mother, the bed-sharing with his parents until he was nine, the childhood games with his cousin, his desire to crash through "the barrier," and his fear of madness; on the other hand, his working life of sacrifice, his care of his family and the economic responsibility, the marriage to Louise, his studies, and the church. These two "lifestyles," which create a constant conflict in Caesar's life, could not be worked through gradually by means of adequate thoughts because of the intensity of the cathexes, which involved opposing loyalties.

Although Caesar leans briefly toward the mother's position at different periods in his life, as when he meets Marianne, reliving the period of bed-sharing or his fantasies with his cousin, his conscious identification with his father's style predominates in his history, although he never relinquishes the other tendency that unconsciously supports the conflict. His sexual development, which coincided with his first migraines, may explain his inclination toward behavior in line with his father's motto: he needed to repress strongly his incestuous tendencies in the wake of the pubertal increase of excitation.

The rational activity that Caesar is able to put to good use for difficult work does not, in spite of appearances, actually constitute a real ability to think adequately with a well-tempered distribution of the cathexes invested in the dilemmas that torture him. In that sense, his thinking still depends on the rationalization of his problems. Thus, he "reasons" that perhaps it was better for Marianne's death to separate them.

While in common headaches an insoluble dilemma (or "inconceivable" problem) remains unconscious and is expressed by the painful ischemic disorder, in Caesar's case the predominance or conscious acceptance of one motto associated with the unconscious persistence of the other one enables us to understand that the hemicranial pain assumes the representation of the consciously omitted motto and of the conflict between the two. The fact that it is on the left side concords with the type of motto omitted, since this motto is associated with the instinct that goes against the norms.

VIII. AN "INCONCEIVABLE" ATTACK

Moses, age 64, had taken a few days' vacation in the mountains with Rebecca. . . . The second night, when they were trying to make love . . . according to what his wife told him, he had the attack. . . . The doctors diagnosed a right hemiplegia, associated with aphasia in recovery (grade III encephalopathy), as sequelae of a cerebrovascular accident, probably a thrombosis. They also found, judging from what he could read in the diagnoses, a hypertensive grade I cardiac disorder, with retinopathy and nephropathy.

He had been suffering from high blood pressure for ten years . . . and sometimes his nose bled. . . . All that started when he was 54. . . . It was a bad period. . . . His mother, he was her favorite, had just died. . . . Israel was at war. . . . Sometimes he had chest pains and his sexual potency had begun to waver. . . .

But the problems dated from before then . . . his life had always been tough. . . . He was the eldest of seven siblings. His father, a pious and strict tanner, used to whip him with his belt for any little thing . . . especially because he resisted going to the Jewish school. . . . They, there in Poland, got along very badly. . . . If it had happened nowadays, Moses thinks, you get a divorce and that's it . . . but at that time, when he had just been born, his mother ran away from their home and only returned several years later.

He was twenty-four when he met Rebecca, a co-worker in his sister Sarah's knitting factory. His first time was when he was eighteen with a prostitute. . . .

He was always very persistent. . . . Whenever he went under commercially, he was able to recover . . . in spite of the renal colics . . . and in spite of the fact that his siblings didn't want to help him. . . . But the resentment, plus his pride about pulling through on his own, stuck in his soul . . . and a sequel of a hernia remained in his body . . . the consequence of a peritonitis he suffered at that time, because of a neglected appendicitis.

He had to separate from Ephraim, his own brother, because he was drawing more money than was his due . . . and two years ago, just when his sons were beginning to gradually take over the management of the business, the gallbladder operation . . . and the accident when he had gone through the windshield . . . and they had had to take him out unconscious, with his right hand injured. . . . But he was always very tenacious . . . and suffered very much. . . .

Last year, a car ran over him when he stepped off the sidewalk, and it was only a miracle that saved him from a fractured skull . . . and again! He got hit in the same arm.

He was in love when he married Rebecca . . . he's always been faithful to her . . . and when he found her with the masseur that summer, in an awkward situation, he couldn't believe it. . . . Now that their last son was married, she had insisted that they leave the big house to move, the two of them alone, to a smaller apartment. But before . . . the trip to the mountains. . . . He had always been very tenacious . . . and suffered very much. . . .

When Moses was trying to make love, he had the attack. Here we clearly see how the cerebrovascular accident, to which the two car accidents were the prelude, takes the place of an unaccomplished action. It is also evident that the action that was substituted is an action that has become conflictual as a result of the contradiction that has taken shape as a dilemma: the strict control of his father or the uncontrolled impulsiveness of his mother.

Moses is replete with an old resentment that is born anew when he discovers his wife's infidelity; however, he does not want to give vent to those violent emotions that would force him to leave her. All to the contrary, he is even afraid that his wife might leave him more permanently than his mother did, since "Nowadays you divorce and that's it." For this reason, paradoxically, when she suggests that the two of them go to live alone in a small apartment, a situation that was rehearsed in the trip to the mountains, he feels that he must always perform "tenaciously" well in bed. However, he feels that achieving performance of this quality is a humiliating submission that leaves his grudges and violent desires for revenge unfulfilled. These same unfulfilled wishes, because of their passionate nature, are the part of the repressed dilemma that is represented by the cerebrovascular accident on the left side.

IX. THE MYTH OF THE BIRTH OF PALLAS ATHENA FROM ZEUS' HEAD

As we indicated in discussing migraine as an inconceivable "disconcertedness" of thought, the word "conceive" means both initiating pregnancy and forming ideas or beginning to feel affects (Real Academia Española, 1950; Corominas, 1961). It is no coincidence that this association between pregnancy and delivery and "gestation of" and "giving birth to" ideas is found frequently in different contexts. We think that this association between the two forms or definitions of conception can be better understood if we recall that in an earlier work (Chiozza, 1970), when we discussed the vicissitudes or manifestations of the "narcissistic" or "metabolic" pregenital organization, we established correlations among growth, procreation, and sublimation. We indicated that sublimation is the creation of forms that are external to the subject. The myth of the birth of Pallas Athena (Minerva) from Zeus' head is perhaps one that most adequately represents this association.

Pallas Athena is the goddess of creativity, wisdom, intelligent reason, and peace. Because she was Zeus' most successful creation, she is nearly his feminine equivalent in mythology, as well as one of his most powerful allies and counselors (Swarthy, 1939; Perez Rioja, 1962).

In the main version of the myth (Swarthy, 1939; Perez Rioja, 1962; Grimal, 1981) Zeus, having conceived an as yet unborn child with Metis (Prudence, Meditation), was given a prophecy announcing that the children he begot with her would surpass or dethrone him. Fearing that the prophecy would be fulfilled, Zeus ate the pregnant Metis. A short time later, he began to suffer terrible pain "in the brain." Hephaestes (Vulcan), the god of fire and the Olympian ironsmith, came to his rescue and, to cure him, split his skull open with an axe. Thus, Athena was born from Zeus' head.

Other versions of the myth (Aeschylus, undated) say that Athena was not gestated by a woman but originated directly from Zeus' head. Considering the symbolic meaning of Athena's attributes, these versions heavily support the impression that the gestation of the goddess expresses and represents the conception and development of ideas.

From our interpretations, we deduce that the deepest or most important interpretation of the myth implies that the "cephalic pregnancy" of Zeus means that ideational capacity, inspiration, the ideal, impregnates or involves meditation and transforms it into a sublimatory process represented in some versions of the myth by the god's own head while in others it is symbolized by the figure of Metis. However, we think that the version of the myth that includes Metis can also be interpreted as a sign of men's jealousy and envy of women's ability to be pregnant and of the relationship between mother and unborn child. While the first interpretation refers to the process of creating ideas, the second alludes to procreation.

We believe that the prophecy to Zeus that he would be surpassed or dethroned by the children he had by Metis represents, in the "procreation" myth, Zeus's own wish to dethrone his father. We think that in the "ideational" version of the myth, the prophecy represents the fantasies and affects that the importance of the ideas inspires and that hinder or prevent their conception.

Zeus' headache symbolizes an inconceivable problem-dilemma constituted by the struggle between the opposing mottos that represent the conflicting affects. One of the mottos expresses his love and his desire to have descendants, whether in the form of ideas or children; the other one represents his possessive and destructive ambitions. In other words, Zeus' conflict represents the struggle between his endangered narcissism and his procreative tendency.

The visual symptoms of migraine (scintillating scotoma and ocular pain) symbolize both the "visual" impact of the ideal forms and the "visual-ideal" component of envy (Chiozza, 1963). Popular sayings refer to this affect with the expression "they gave him the evil eye"; resentment and vengeance are warded off with the toast, "Here's mud in your eye."

When affects are very intense, they bring along a component of action that disturbs or impedes the development of the subject's creative (sublimatory) capacity. When impulsive, primary "acting" is generated, these affects impede the normal and adequate development of the thought process that enables achievement of adequate thought representations and moderate external actions. This impulsive action is represented in the myth by the devouring of pregnant Metis: Zeus is overwhelmed by extremely violent emotions and is forced to annul or to "abort" the ideas or descendants in order to prevent their development.

Hephaestes, the god of fire and its personification, is at the same time the divine blacksmith and is characterized as the most hard-working and industrious of the inhabitants of Olympus (Perez Rioja, 1962). When he splits Zeus' head open with his axe, he makes Athena's birth possible. This symbolizes the predominance of the procreative impulse: the ego's "hepatic" capacity, the strength, experience, and the will of the ego, that allow "the knot hindering development of ideas to be untied" and children to be conceived.

X. The Myth of Orestes

The struggle between passion and reason is represented in the Oresteia (Aeschylus, undated). Orestes must resolve a serious conflict: he must obey the command of the god Apollo to avenge the death of his father, Agamemnon, who was murdered by his mother, Clytaemnestra. The choice, the "inconceivable problem-dilemma," is either to kill his mother in order to avenge his father's death or to protect her and thus leave his father's death unpunished. Orestes decides to act according to one of his mottos: to obey the command of Apollo, who says that the father is more important than the mother and that if he does not carry out the revenge, great ills will befall his people and himself.

After killing Clytaemnestra, Orestes is pursued by the Furies (the unnamable one, vengeful destruction and rancor), goddesses who punish crimes against mothers with torture and madness. As a consequence of the punishment, Orestes is left alone for several days in great pain with his head and eyes covered (Graves, 1960; Perez Rioja, 1962).

The laws governing the representation of dreams (Freud, 1900a, p. 339) can also be applied to the interpretation of myths; therefore, we can reason that the torture and madness inflicted by the Furies symbolically condense, by an inversion of time or a decomposition of the conflict into two moments, that of the crime and that of repentance, Orestes' contradictory passions before choosing one of his mottos. We can accept this interpretation if we remember that the description of the hero's suffering is very similar to the symptoms of a migraine attack.

X. Summary of Vascular Headache and Cerebrovascular Accidents as Specific Unconscious Fantasies

1. The clinical form of migraine called "migraine with complications" involves persistent organic alterations ranging from cerebral edema to the permanent sequelae of ischemia. Drawing an analogy with what occurs between the angina pectoris and the cardiac infarct, we infer a series of gradual transitions from the vascular headaches to the cerebral infarcts.

2. The thought processes on the one hand and the representations of brain and head on the other enter consciousness from the same unconscious dispositional structure. We assume that the brain or encephalon intervenes preponderantly in thinking and that, consequently, the brain (or the head) usually represents the thought processes.

3. By small, tentative cathexes, the thought processes contribute to configuring the different models of action. "Effective actions" are those that succeed in putting an end to the need that comes from the drive source. However, an action is appropriate when, regardless of its efficacy, its meaning is comprehensible and it is directed toward an aim. Since the affects or discharge processes with "full" cathexes are the persistence in the present of phylogenetically expedient actions, thought can be used for tempering the affects.

4. The need to temper the affects arises when conflict is generated by contradictory emotions. Then, the discharge of the cathexes, which occurs according to the norm or innervation key qualifying an affect, hypercathects the innervation key of another one or impedes its discharge, acting as a countercathexis.

With regard to the degree to which affects can be tempered, we distinguish passions (primary affects) from feelings (secondary affects) and from impassive words stripped of emotion.

5. A "motto" is a principle of action, held as a product of a preformed judgment (prejudice), that consciously or unconsciously orients behavior. Since the affects are processes discharged according to phylogenetically appropriate norms of action, mottos can be considered cogitative equivalents of the affects. Therefore, they can be used for tempering the affects. When this is accomplished, emotions are discharged

by means of moderate and adequate words and actions. When the emotional conflict continues because it is represented in coexisting and yet opposing mottos, the subject is faced with a dilemma.

6. The dilemma may eventually become a rational problem in which each motto is examined and revalued in relation to its opposite; further, we can consider the present circumstances involved in the conflict that determine variations in the applicability of each of them. But when the mottos involved in the conversion of a dilemma into a problem function as rationalizations that fail to temper the subjacent affects they represent, an insoluble problem-dilemma takes shape. The situation can then be described in the words of Pascal: "The heart has reasons that reason ignores." It can then be said that the patient intends to treat an emotional conflict that remains unconscious as if it were a rational problem that makes the person impassive. This happens when the subject's previous attempt to transform the emotional conflict into an authentic rational problem through an adequate "cogitative" representation has failed. Because of its capacity for tempering the affects, this representation would have allowed thought to operate with small cathexes in resolving the conflict.

7. Since we can assume that the cerebral vascular processes are part of the normal "innervation key" of the thought processes, we can safely say that the vascular headache (and the ischemic cerebral disorder it involves) is an equivalent manifestation, both expressive and symbolic, of a problem-dilemma that has become insoluble. Instead of producing a pathosomatic decomposition of the "innervation key" of the affects involved in the present conflict, as occurs in other circumstances, the "innervation keys" of the thought constituting the dilemma or the problem representing those affects cogitatively lose their coherence. Thus, the dilemma or problem fails to enter consciousness, or enters it only partly, and the headache occurs in its place.

The headaches manifested as a throbbing pain are the most typical representation of their unconscious meaning, since in these cases the head "throbs" as if it were a heart. The often-heard expression in Spanish, "the blood went to my head," owes its origin to the formerly conscious perception of the fantasies involved in the headache.

8. The cogitative representation of an emotional conflict that has not been represented in a dilemma or in a problem constitutes the cogitative "disconcertedness" which we term "inconceivable." When this situation reaches consciousness, the subject usually says, "I don't know what to think" or "I can't get it into my head."

The specific unconscious meanings of the ischemic cerebral disorder whose clinical manifestation is migraine depend on the mosaic of fantasies that configure the set of its most frequent symptoms: hemicrania, scintillating scotomas, ocular pain, nausea, and vomiting. The intensity of the pain, usually exceeding that of common headache, could very well be constituted as a deformation of the innervation key of the cogitative processes that have been unable to overcome the "disconcertedness" in order to achieve the configuration of a dilemma.

Scintillating scotomas, photophobia, and ocular pain in migraine seem to adequately represent the "visual" traumatic impact of some ideal forms, whose meaning the word "dazzling" evokes. Nausea and vomiting reveal a "hepatic" failure in the task of materializing or assimilating these ideal demands. As for the hemicrania that is clinically difficult to explain, it links the symptoms of vascular headaches with those of the cerebrovascular accidents that evolve with hemiplegia. It probably symbolically expresses one of the mottos in conflict.

9. Any thought, however weak the cathexis of its representations may be, always involves a motor discharge. All motor discharges are constituted from the sum of an emotional vegetative component, discharged in the body, added to an action component that is discharged in relation to the objects of the world. The cogitative process configures the norms of action that are preserved in unconscious memory as norms of effective action, once they have proved to be so by the experience that put them into action. Thus, this process goes through a series of stages ranging from the ideas and judgments involved in imprecise, vacillating, impulsive, or tentative movements to those of the most elaborate and precise motor coordinations. Thought and action are thus indissolubly united in the unconscious—not only because the omnipotence of ideas governing the unconscious psyche considers them equivalent, but also because the "innervation key" of the thought processes is closely connected to the "innervation key" of the motor acts of relational life— just as closely as the functions of thought and experience are.

10. When the intensity of the affects that motivate cogitative activity is transferred to relations with objects of the real world, we say that thought is "enacted" or that it is associated with a "high" component of action, this meaning that action prematurely "interrupts" thought. In this case, both the dilemma and the "disconcertedness" arising from an intense emotional conflict lead to the experience of a conflict of actions or a sensory-motor "disconcertedness"—conflict and "disconcertedness" that take shape, respectively, as indecision and motor powerlessness. Because of the unconscious equivalency between thought and action, the inconceivable and the impossible reinforce each other.

11. We believe that it is mainly the brain or encephalon that intervenes in thinking and that the cerebral vascular processes are part of the "innervation key" of the thought processes. Since the brain functions as a "center" directing the sensory-motor activity that configures actions, we infer that these vascular processes are also part of the "innervation key" of actions. We can therefore say that the ischemic disorders translated into an edema or a cerebral infarct, which transiently or permanently annul the sensory-motor functions, are the expressive and symbolic equivalent of a

cogitative "disconcertedness" or dilemma that involves a large component of action. This dilemma or "disconcertedness" has remained unconscious, transferring "the whole" of its full cathexis to the cerebral
vascular–parenchymatous process that is normally part of the "innervation key" of the actions involved, thus transforming them into a "somatic"
disorder.

The involvement of an action component in the alterations of thought
hidden in cerebrovascular accidents not only enables us to understand the
sensory-motor involvement, whose diverse clinical forms correlate with
the different actions involved, but also their customary occurrence as a
sudden ictus or stroke that leads us to call them "accidents."

8

ORGANSPRACHE: A REVISION OF THE FREUDIAN CONCEPT[1]

L. A. CHIOZZA

> Freud used the term *Organsprache* in his paper on "The unconscious" (1915e, p. 198) to refer to a concept he intertwined throughout his works, from "Studies on hysteria" (Freud & Breuer, 1895d) to "An outline of psychoanalysis" (Freud, 1940a).

I. ON LANGUAGE AND SPEECH

In his English translation of Freud's works, Strachey used the compound noun "organ-speech" for the term *Organsprache*. However, both López Ballesteros and Etcheverry, the two translators of Freud into Spanish, use the word *lenguaje* (language), perhaps because Spanish has no term etymologically akin to the German *Sprache* like the English word "speech" (Partridge, 1966; Skeat, 1882) (Fig. 1). The Spanish *lenguaje*, deriving from *lengua* (tongue), originally designated speech as a faculty and as a means of expression effected by vocal sounds. Its meaning later broadened to include any sign system, with or without the actual formation of sound (Real Academia Española, 1950; *Enciclopedia Salvat*, 1985). In English, as in Italian and in French, equivalents of the word *lenguaje* can be traced back to the same etymological root. This is not the case in German, where the meaning,

---

[1]The text of this chapter is derived from a paper presented at a seminar on *Organsprache*, held in Rome in July 1989 with the participation of André Green.

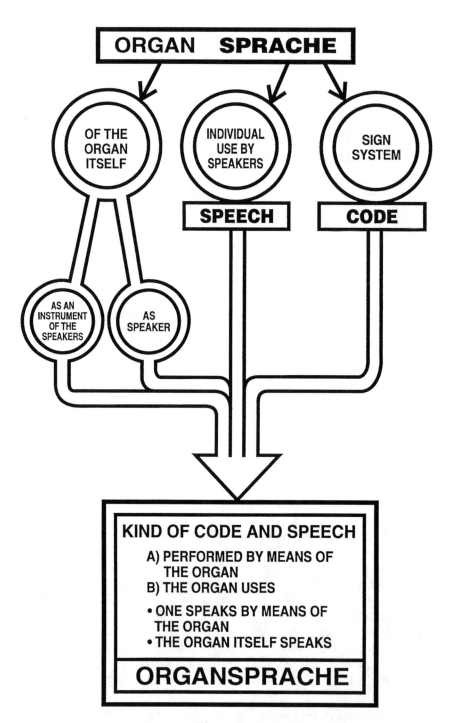

Figure 1

"sign system," included in the Spanish word *lenguaje*, is conveyed by *Sprache*, which is not derived from *Zunge* (tongue). For example, written language is *Schriftsprache*, spoken language, *Lautsprache*, expressive language, *Expressivsprache*, the language of the eyes, *Augensprache*, and sign language, *Zeichensprache*. We may conclude that in Spanish, either Etcheverry's phrase, *lenguaje de órgano* or López Ballesteros' *lenguaje de los órganos* translates the German word well if it is clear that in these phrases the word *lenguaje* designates not only a sign system but also means, both directly and figuratively, the Spanish *habla* (speech): the individual use of a language by its speakers[2] (de Saussure, 1945). Freud undoubtedly had this definition of *Organsprache* in mind. In his case history of "Dora" (1905e), describing a symptomatic act in which Dora gestured with her hands, he asserted that "no mortal can keep a secret. If his lips are silent, he chatters with his finger-tips; betrayal oozes out of him at every pore" (1905e, pp. 77–78).

II. The Organ Speaks

In "The unconscious" (1915e), in discussing language disturbances in schizophrenia, Freud referred to one of Tausk's patients who described her ailments, complaining that "her eyes were not right, they were twisted" (Freud, 1915e, p. 198). It was the patient's particular way of representing the vicissitudes of a quarrel she had had with her lover, whom she considered an "eye-twister" (*Augenverdreher*, a deceiver). The same patient reported that "She was standing in church. Suddenly she felt a jerk; she had to change her position, as though somebody was putting her into a position," thus expressing the idea that her lover "had placed her in a false position." With regard to the former example, Freud agreed with Tausk that "the patient's relation to a bodily organ (the eye) has arrogated to itself the representation of the whole content" and added, "Here the schizophrenic utterance exhibits a hypochondriacal trait: it has become '*organ speech*.'" A few lines further on, he stated that the two utterances of this patient "argue in favour of what we have called hypochondriacal speech or 'organ speech'" (Freud, 1915e, p. 198).

This is the starting point for a basic problem. Since the schizophrenic utterance is a verbal statement, a cursory reading of Freud could lead us to believe that in "hypochondriacal language" or "organ language," a particular organ becomes the referent (or grammatical subject) of a verbal phrase or discourse. In that case, the patient would be talking about an organ and would be doing it with words. However, closer reading enables us to understand that, in the paragraph quoted, when Freud

---

[2] In F. de Saussure's sense of the word *parole*, similar to N. Chomsky's concept of "performance."

mentioned the hypochrondriacal trait exhibited by the schizophrenic utterance, he was alluding to a more complex way of thinking.

1. On the same page, Freud stated that a hysterical patient would have actually twisted her eyes convulsively or (in the second example) would have actually jerked—i.e., she would not have expressed herself in a verbal language. This, he added, would have taken place instead of "having the *impulse* to do so or the *sensation* of doing so" (Freud, 1915e, p. 198). It seems evident that this somatic sensation is the "hypochrondriacal trait" to which Freud alluded.

2. Moreover, the grammatical form of the compound noun "organ-speech" leaves no doubt that here "organ" indicates the kind of speech one is talking about (Eckersley, 1960). Likewise, the examination of many examples similar to the one we have quoted certifies that the same is true of the German term *Organsprache*. Accordingly, it refers to a special kind of language, the language "of the organ," which is different from verbal language. Therefore, Freud's writings imply that schizophrenic utterance which is verbal is not yet organ-speech but may exhibit the character of this type of speech when it shows a "hypochondriacal trait." That is, whether through a perceptible somatic change (a sign), as in hysteria, or through a somatic sensation (a symptom), as in hypochondria, one speaks by means of the organ—or the organ itself speaks, as we shall see later.

The idea not only that verbal discourse may have as referents the organs and their functions but also that the organs themselves may "join in the conversation" (*mitsprechen*) are already present in Anna O.'s case history (Freud & Breuer, 1895d). The term *mitsprechen*, denoting "the interesting and not undesired phenomenon" (Freud, 1895b) by which a symptom, sensation, or disturbance "responds," "interferes," "intervenes," "takes part," or "joins in the conversation" reappears in several of Freud's works (1895d, p. 37; 1896b, 1918b).

III. The Erotogenic Zone as Source, Agent, and Object of Linguistic Expression

In a dense and lengthy paragraph of Elisabeth von R.'s case history (1895d) discussing symbolization in hysteria, Freud examined the current usage of some verbal expressions: the equation of being insulted with receiving "a slap in the face" (Freud & Breuer, 1895d, p. 178), of being slighted with feeling "a stab in the heart" (1895d, p. 180), of being unable to return an insult with "having to swallow it" (1895d, p. 180). He went on to say that if we had not already experienced those specific bodily sensations at some time in the past in the same circumstances that the affects alluded to, we would never have invented these verbal expressions. In these cases, Freud remarked, the verbal expression seems "only a figurative picture" because the physical sensations and innervations accompanying and expressing those emotions have become greatly weakened, though they originally "had a meaning and served a purpose," as Darwin taught us.

On this basis, Freud concluded that "hysteria is right in restoring the original meaning of the words in depicting its unusually strong innervations" (Freud & Breuer, 1895d, p. 181) when it revives "the sensations to which the verbal expression owes its justification." And he suggested that perhaps the hysterical symptom ". . . *does not take linguistic usage as its model at all, but that both hysteria and linguistic usage draw their material from a common source.*" Thus, one source, identifiable as the erotogenic zone where a drive has originated, reaches consciousness as a somatic sensation (e.g., a dysphagia) on the one hand, while on the other hand it cathects the preconscious word-presentations forming the verbal expression or figure of speech (to have "to swallow" an insult, in this case).

Freud (1905d) made it clear that erogenization, following the paths of mutual influence, disturbs the physiological function that is part of the unconscious innervation key (Freud, 1900a) of a normal affect. However, in the case we are discussing, what also happens is that the unusual innervations and inhibitions constituting the physical symptoms of hysteria are the transposition of a normal affect that has been "strangled" because it has developed in a pathogenic situation. "When the bed of a stream is divided into two channels, then, if the current in one of them is brought up against an obstacle, the other will at once be overfilled" (Freud, 1910a, p. 18).

It is noteworthy that aside from the two paths mentioned above (the somatic sensation and the cathexis of preconscious presentations), there is a third one in which excitation is discharged in a totally unconscious way while modifying physical structure or function. In the latter case, the sense organs or their instrumental extensions sometimes perceive its effects as a somatic change unassociated with any sensation (Fig. 2–5).

These three pathways (perception of a somatic change, somatic sensations, and preconscious representations) through which excitation arising from the source of a drive reaches consciousness coincide with the three ways in which excitation at a source may be produced, in Freud's view: from the external world, from inside the body, or from psychical life (Freud, 1905d). We understand how this coincidence "closes a circle" between the "centrifugal" and "centripetal" directions of excitation when we realize that the psychoanalytic theory of the erotogenic zones (which originated in the previous concept of hysterogenous zones) implies that each zone may be the source, the object, and also the agent of drive excitation. Therefore, when the subject speaks about an organ, and more so, when the subject speaks by

ORIGIN OF THE FIGURE OF SPEECH

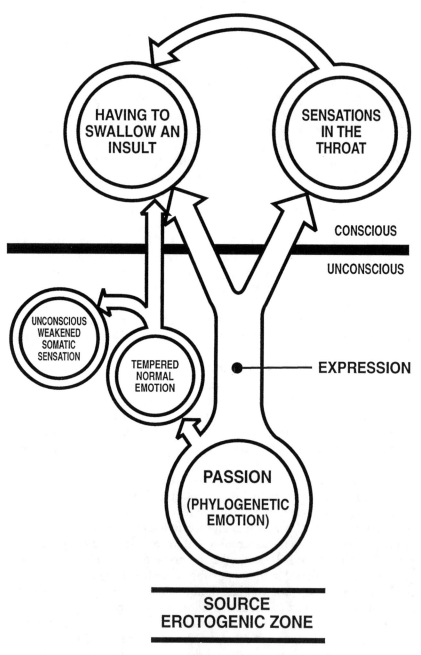

Figure 2

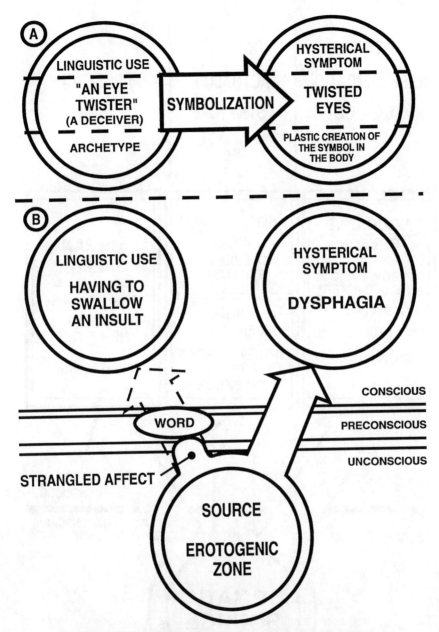

WHEN THE HYSTERICAL SYMPTOM SEEMS TO BE
TAKING THE FIGURE OF SPEECH AS AN ARCHETYPE (A),
THEN BOTH ARE ACTUALLY DRAWING THEIR MATERIAL
FROM A COMMON SOURCE (B)

Figure 3

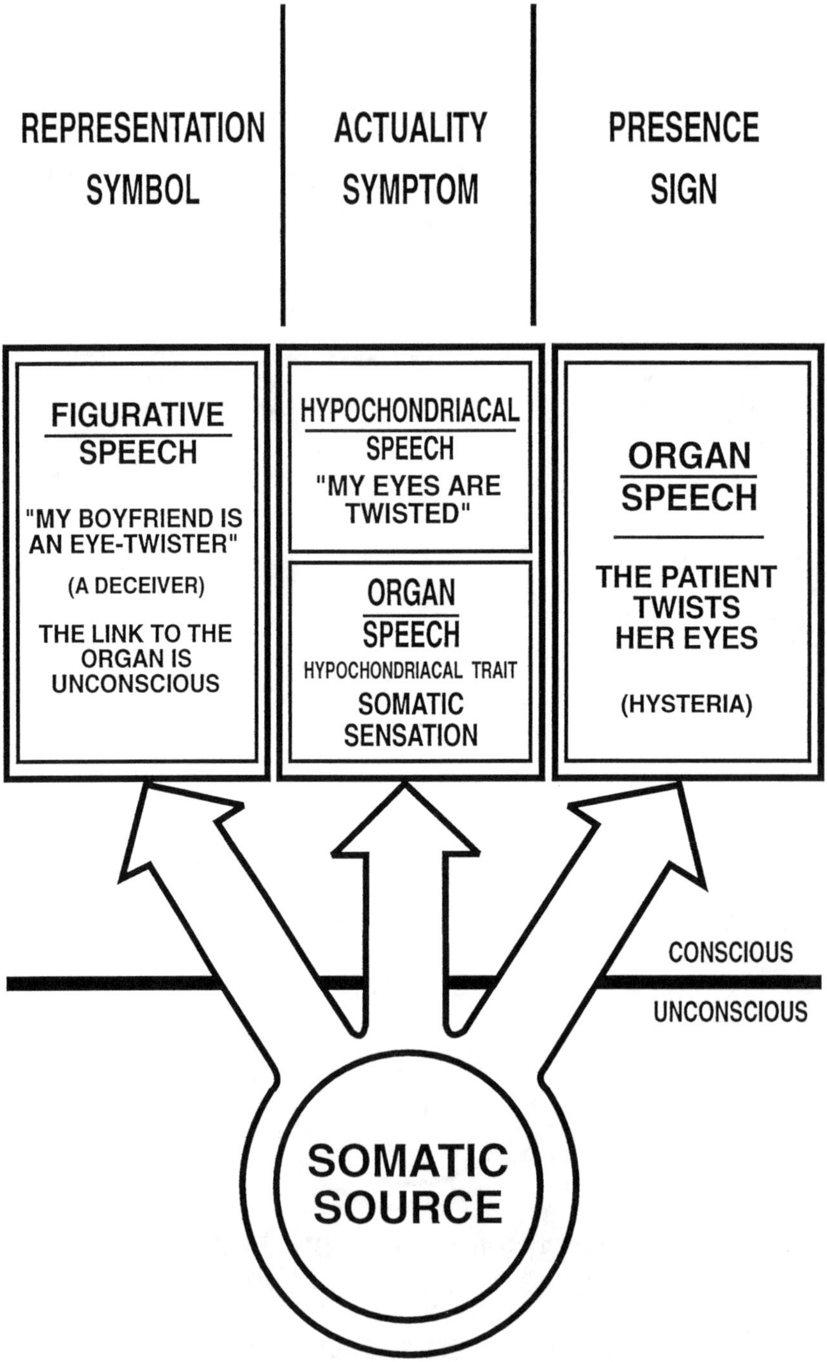

REPRESENTATION SYMBOL	ACTUALITY SYMPTOM	PRESENCE SIGN
FIGURATIVE SPEECH "MY BOYFRIEND IS AN EYE-TWISTER" (A DECEIVER) THE LINK TO THE ORGAN IS UNCONSCIOUS	HYPOCHONDRIACAL SPEECH "MY EYES ARE TWISTED" **ORGAN SPEECH** HYPOCHONDRIACAL TRAIT SOMATIC SENSATION	**ORGAN SPEECH** THE PATIENT TWISTS HER EYES (HYSTERIA)

CONSCIOUS

UNCONSCIOUS

SOMATIC SOURCE

Figure 4

ORGAN SPEECH

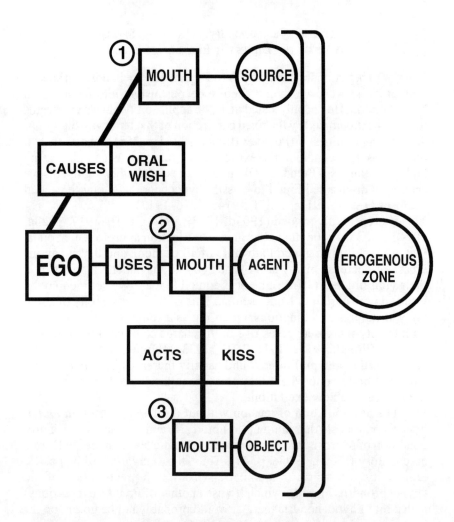

(1) THE MOUTH SPEAKS WITH THE EGO ACT

(2) THE EGO ACT SPEAKS WITH THE MOUTH

(3) THE EGO ACT SPEAKS OF THE OBJECT MOUTH

Figure 5

means of an organ, it is the organ itself that is speaking. Since it is grounded in primary meanings, the wish directed by "the subject" toward a mouth (object), or *the desire expressed with the mouth (agent), is an oral wish that the mouth (source) "makes" the subject express.*

IV. HYPOCHONDRIACAL SPEECH AND THE SPECIFIC AIMS OF THE DIFFERENT EROTOGENIC ZONES

In order to better understand why Freud equated hypochondriacal speech with organ-speech, we should acquire deeper insight into his ideas on hypochondria. He not only stated that "the applicability of its name seems to me to be prejudiced by the fixed connection of that term with the symptom of 'fear of illness'" (Freud & Breuer, 1895d, p. 258), but also that "it requires as a precondition the existence of paraesthesias and distressing bodily sensations" (Freud, 1895b, p. 93). These and other arguments we shall now discuss led Freud to classify hypochondria among the actual neuroses (1895b, 1911c, 1912f, 1914c, 1916–1917).

He repeatedly argued (1905d, 1913j, 1914c, 1916–1917, 1923a, 1924c, 1933a, 1940a) that all organs can function as erotogenic zones, that erogeneity is a general attribute of all of them, and that it can increase or decrease in any part of the body. In his paper, "Instincts and their vicissitudes" (1915c), he also argued that a drive source may be inferred with certainty from its aims. This specific erogeneity of some body structures and functions, emerging as a somatic sensation when its intensity increases, gives rise on discharge to organ-pleasure (*Organlust*) (Freud, 1915c, 1916–1917, 1933a). Organ-pleasure is autoerotic, partial, and preliminary and usually increases libidinal tension since the body zone where that pleasure is discharged then becomes the source of a new excitation.

The accumulation of tension without discharge creates an *actual* hypochrondriacal "damming up of libido" (Freud, 1914c, p. 85), a precondition of neurosis that Freud named "somatic compliance" in Dora's case history (Freud, 1905e, p. 41). Thus, the *"actuality"* of a specific erogeneity gives birth to a somatic sensation, a precondition of the "hypochrondriacal trait," which (to use another of Freud's expressions) is that bit of hypochondria that, "it would probably not be going too far to suppose," is part of any neurosis (1914c, p. 83).

A second basic problem arises at this point: in the light of Freud's own concept of hypochrondriacal speech, the opposition between "actuality" and "meaning" deriving from the classification of neuroses into actual neuroses and psychoneuroses, or into what Freud (1910i) called neurotic and psychogenic organ disorders, cannot be supported, since speech is meaning. According to his own statements, there is a bit of hypochondria, and an actual component with it, in any psychoneurosis. Furthermore, again according to Freud, the amount of excitation determining the "actuality" is always connected to a specific feature, that is, with an aim, end, sense, or meaning. It is notable that the expression "hypochondriacal speech" conveys two meanings: the actuality of the hypochondria and the meaning of speech. On the other hand, the usefulness and validity of the concept of "actuality" is beyond doubt. It is a basic component of psychoanalytic theory that is present all along, beginning with the distinction between perception and memory (or between sign and symbol), and going on to the metapsychology of affect and of efficient action (Fig. 6). If we go back to the idea that perception, sensation, and memory constitute the three "origins" of the "contents" of the unconscious, we must differentiate: (1) the "physical" presence that is perceived by the sensory organs as being a "fact" of the world whose source is in the past; (2) the "historical" actuality that arises as the "psychical" sensation of an event that is occurring in the body itself, or of an act that is taking place in that same body; (3) the "atemporal" representation of a memory-wish that takes the "spiritual" form of a meaning, of an ideal and future aim; (4) physical absence, which is constituted when what is remembered or desired is not perceived; (5) historical latency, constituted when what is represented is experienced as postponement or waiting because it lacks the conscious "somatic" sensation belonging to an event taking place; and (6) the incoherence of meaning that is constituted when an actual sensation lacks a conscious aim or meaning.

V. The Code in Which The Organ Speaks

The discussion of the issues raised by organ-speech leads us to the subject of archaic inheritance. Freud dealt with the continuity between phylogeny and ontogeny in several texts, for example, in his discussion of the universal symbol (1900a, 1916–1917), of the primal fantasy (1916–1917, 1918b), and of the analogy between hysteria as an individual, newly formed affect and the affect as a generalized hysteria which has been inherited and contains the reminiscence of a phylogenetic event (1926d, 1933a). Since erotogenic zones give rise to drives whose specific aims enable us to infer their sources,[3] the particular feature of a drive aim has a *specific relationship* with a definite part of the structure and functioning of the body. To say that a relationship is specific means that the "preferential" link of one of its terms with the other is "universal," inasmuch as it is shared by all other similar organisms.

---

[3]Although instincts are wholly determined by their origin in a somatic source, in mental life we know them only by their aims . . . [S]ometimes [an instinct's] source may be inferred from its aim. [Freud 1915c, p. 123]

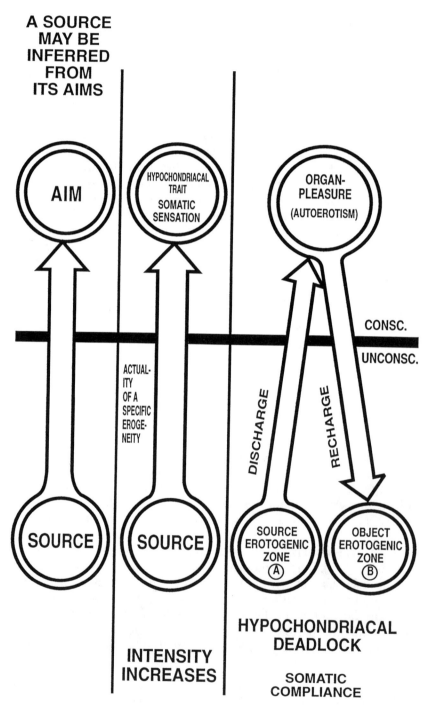

Figure 6

Some changes in the structure and functioning of a part of the body constitute organ-speech, given that such universality is equivalent to sharing a code or a sign system. One of the most frequent examples of those relationships is the link between blushing and shame, which is organically determined and therefore universally shared. Hence, organ-speech is as universal as the inborn symbols kept alive in myths, dreams, figures of speech, and art. Freud even told us of "an old and extinct way of expression, many elements of which have been kept alive in different areas," linking it to Schreber's idea of a fundamental language that leaves some symbolic references as lasting residues (1911c).

In his paper, "The claims of psychoanalysis to scientific interest" (1913j), Freud stated that ". . . the unconscious speaks more than one dialect," again addressing the idea of a language using the same figurative resources one finds in dreams (1900a) and able to express a given meaning by different means. When Freud took the model of somatic compliance to signal the existence of a "linguistic compliance" (1901b), he made it clear that the latter not only enables us to improve our definition of the event we seek to interpret (a slip of the tongue or of the pen) but also determines its limits.

On this basis, and on the basis of the idea that the physical symptom "joins in the conversation," Weizsaecker (1956) built his concept of "organ-dialect." According to Weizsaecker (1956, p. 210), each organ uses its own "speech" to participate in the "chorus of voices"; but he added that what Freud (1900a) called "consideration of representability" (only what can be "represented" as a picture can be dreamt) also applies in this case. The richness of each organ's vocabulary is determined by its structure and function. Each organ has its own "dialect," its unique and specific linguistic code, composed of a few "words" which define its way of speaking.

However, were these the only alternatives, organ-speech would be too poor to account for the particular meanings belonging to each erotogenic zone. A "strangled" affect may reach discharge by hypercathexis of some of the unique innervations belonging to its normal key. The relatively awkward code of an organ-dialect recovers its full wealth of meaning precisely from its "latent" capacity to evoke the meaning of the key that has been distorted by the defensive process in the interpreter. In the patient's unconscious, the symptom through which the cathexis is discharged has become the compromise, the symbolic representative of the emotions involved.

Freud said (1915b) that the genuine aim of repression is the suppression of the development of the affect. Therefore, the affect is the essence of the meaning. The physical symptom that represents an affect involved in a conflict not only "speaks": its meaning is what "tells" us most (Fig. 7).

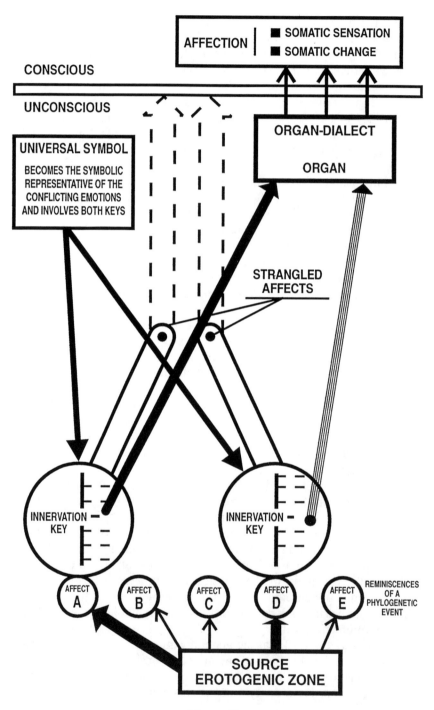

Figure 7

VI. THE SECOND FUNDAMENTAL HYPOTHESIS
OF PSYCHOANALYSIS

When Freud argued, in an early work (1900a), that dreams can be interpreted, he noted that science holds that "the dream is not a psychical act at all, but a somatic process which announces itself in the psychical apparatus through a certain number of signs." In 1915, Freud wrote "Justification for the Concept of the Unconscious" in his paper "The Unconscious" (1915e, p. 166), where he advocates the legitimacy of sustaining the existence of an unconscious psyche. Twenty-five years later he returned to the same discussion, stating that the consensus is that conscious processes do not form closed or unbroken sequences. Therefore, it is assumed "that there are physical or somatic processes which are concomitant with the psychical ones and which we should necessarily have to recognize as more complete than the psychical sequences, since some of them would have conscious processes parallel to them but others would not" (1940a). In another work published in the same year, he remarked that "the equation of what is mental with what is conscious had the unwelcome result of divorcing psychical processes from the general context of events in the universe . . . ," but "the fact could no longer be overlooked that psychical phenomena are to a high degree dependent upon somatic influences and on their side have the most powerful effects upon somatic processes" (1940b, p. 283). The philosophers "were obliged to assume that there were organic processes parallel to the conscious psychical ones, related to them in a manner that was hard to explain. . . . But this solution remained unsatisfactory."

Freud was eighty-two at that time, and it was the last time he was to make a public presentation of his ideas, as Strachey says. His aim was "to bring together the tenets of psychoanalysis in the most unequivocal terms" (1940a, p. 144). He postulated "the second fundamental hypothesis" of psychoanalysis, which "explains the supposedly somatic concomitant phenomena as being what is truly psychical, and thus in the first instance disregards the quality of consciousness" (1940a, p. 158). In other words, we can infer from the second hypothesis that the genuinely psychical has two forms of presenting itself in consciousness. One of them is that which we know as the psychological conscious, the other acquires the form of processes (the alleged somatic concomitant ones) which are somatic only consciously, since, unconsciously, they constitute that which Freud calls the genuinely psychical. This is to say that we consider somatic what is unconsciously and "genuinely" psychical when the meaning that includes it in an unbroken sequence remains unconscious.

This hypothesis processes the most fundamental significance since it not only proves that psychoanalysis is the interpretation of the somatic but also reveals a Freudian epistemology that is generally latent, different from the epistemology we find in many of the concepts he used when he theorized on his discoveries. The author of "The psychoanalytic view of the psychogenic disturbance of vision" (1910i), the man who asserted the existence of a psychical representative of somatic excitation, is very different from the Freud who stated the second fundamental hypothesis: while in the first two theoretical formulations soma and psyche "exist" beyond consciousness, the last one considers them categories that consciousness establishes when it comes into contact with the "thing-in-itself," incomprehensible and not susceptible to categorization as either psychical or somatic.

VII. ORGAN-SPEECH IN THE PSYCHOANALYTIC SESSION

Since organ language has an unconscious meaning, it is material to be interpreted during the psychoanalytic session. We have already differentiated three possibilities: one speaks about the organ or by means of it, or the organ itself speaks. Although the first case lacks organ-speech as such, it is implicit, since the patient speaks of an organ in the analytic session only when the organ "speaks" to him/her. In a passage of his "Psychology of dream processes" (1900a), revised and corrected several times, Freud differentiated psychical from material reality. It was a basic distinction from the very beginning of his work, when he coined the concept of "objective reality signs" (1950a [written in 1895]), up to his latest articles (1940a), where it was associated with the idea of a "disavowal of perceptions." In "A metapsychological complement to the theory of dreams" (1917d), Freud contended that the difference between the way the individual defends himself against the stimuli of the external world and the way he defends himself against excitation deriving from the drives is a distinctive reality sign. Moreover, in a footnote to that same article, Freud differentiated between "reality-testing" and "actuality-testing," though unfortunately he never returned to this subject.

From this perspective, we can distinguish three types of referents in the patient's verbal discourse. He may speak of present things, including his own body, which he perceives in the world; he may speak of his actual somatic sensations; finally, he may also speak of the absence of the former or of the latter, which in the last analysis is the same as speaking of representations. The representations of an organ may cover a wide range that includes, for instance, his knowledge of that organ or the narration of a dream that refers to it (1917d, p. 233).

In metapsychological terms, we may say that these three basic referents of discourse—perceptions, sensations, and memories—are also the basic referents of any kind of language and at the same time the origin of everything entering into consciousness. They come together in a generally unconscious way, giving rise to thoughts, feelings, and intentions.

The "pure" conscious representations are "absences" and "latencies": the cathexes of mnemic traces that reach consciousness by way of their link to perceptual mnemic residues, which are mainly word-representations. The "pure" somatic sensations are actual discharges deriving from the unconscious innervation keys of the affects; like them, they may reach consciousness without necessarily linking to word-representations. The "pure" physical alterations, lacking associated somatic sensations, take place when the discharge of the drive cathexes that modify physical structure or functioning is unconscious.

News of an alteration in the world around or in the subject's body, arriving by way of the five senses, is a presence that depends on how attention selects perceptions; this selection is determined by the specific cathexes of unconscious drives. When things do not happen this way and the alteration is not perceived, this news may instead be received as information obtained from the world by means of preconscious verbal representations. An example is the information acquired from a medical diagnosis (Figs. 8 and 9). In both cases, when a "pure" somatic alteration reaches consciousness, it does so in the form of an "external" perception.

The "pure" somatic alterations (signs) and the somatic sensations deprived of affective meaning (symptoms) are understood by the individual experiencing them as the result of a foreign cause or influence. In the psychoanalytic session, the basic referents we have discussed are evidenced in four ways: (1) in verbal discourse; (2) in other kinds of sensory perception that enable the analyst to detect signs such as pallor, obesity, sweaty hands, etc.; (3) in nonverbal language, including the extrasystemic connotations of language itself, seen in combinations of gestures, behavior, and attitudes; and (4) in all that emerges in the countertransference, the true "power plant" that generates attribution of meaning.

VIII. ORGAN-SPEECH IN TRANSFERENCE AND COUNTERTRANSFERENCE

When Freud described transference for the first time (Freud & Breuer, 1895d), he emphasized that it was a "false link." The patient's compulsion to associate linked the content of the unconscious wish that became conscious during treatment to Freud as a person, with which the patient could rightfully deal. Some time later (1900a), Freud explained this mechanism in metapsychological terms: the unconscious representation, unable to become conscious, transfers its intensity upon a preconscious representation that disguises it and thus becomes undeservedly important. In Dora's case history (1905e), Freud mentioned the difficulties caused by the substitution of "an earlier person by the person of the physician" (1905e, p. 116). Therefore, a transference of "false connection" is created

CONSCIOUS PSYCHOLOGY INTERPRETATION

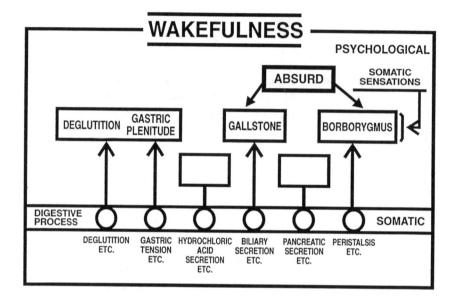

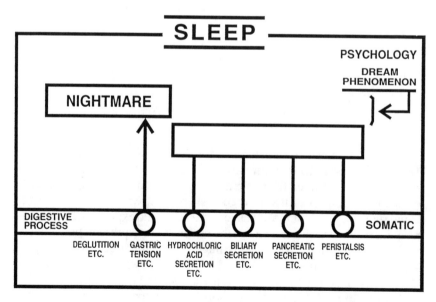

Figure 8

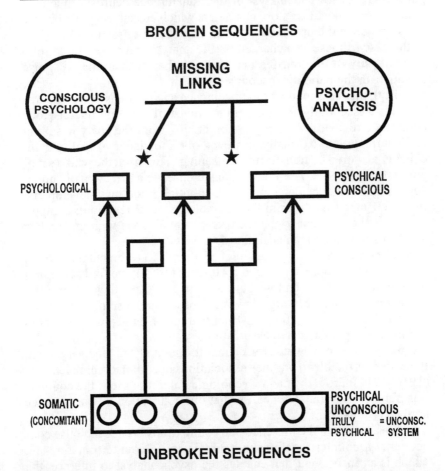

Figure 9

in an "atemporal present," since only the preconscious representation of the psychoanalyst has the signs of reality that differentiate perception from memory in the course of the session (Fig. 10).

The transference neurosis contains the history of the patient's relationship with the analyst, intertwining false links with "real" contacts, since the analyst is also to some extent a real character in the patient's real life. The analyst of the transference neurosis functions in the session like those story characters which are subject to an intense transference in the present—e.g., Mr. K. in Dora's case history. Since in the case of these two characters (the analyst and Mr. K.), the relative intensity of the transference varies, either of them may disguise the other in the patient's discourse.

Both the false connection transference and the transference neurosis derive essentially from the transference of infantile unconscious complexes revived by the regression arising from the analytic setting and interpretation. Normally, however, our knowledge of reality is inevitably acquired by transferring a meaning taken from the whole set of our past experiences. This kind of transference, which is a tool of knowledge, cannot be considered neurotic, although it too may develop and free itself increasingly from the components of its repetition compulsion; it is the one that forms the therapeutic alliance with the analyst and helps to maintain an adequate setting.

The potential countertransference offers as a technical instrument have been thoroughly examined by Racker (1958); we find some precedents in Freud. He had written not only that ". . . the doctor's unconscious is able, from the derivatives of the unconscious which are communicated to him, to reconstruct that unconscious, which has determined the patient's free associations" (1912f, p. 116), but also legitimized the use of whatever occurs to the analyst, precisely when the patient is unable to produce associations to certain dream elements (1916–1917). From the metapsychological point of view, the countertransference is a transference, so that our conception of transference applies to it as well.

We are then in the presence of a countertransference of "false connection," a countertransference neurosis and a countertransference, which is an instrument that enables the psychoanalyst to interpret the repressed unconscious in the patient. Racker had the merit of showing that the first two forms of countertransference can also be converted into technical instruments if utilized appropriately. As for the way in which organ-speech emerges in the transference–countertransference, the following may be asserted:

1. "Pure" conscious representations, which are "absences," tend to be transferred onto the characters in the patient's narration; these characters include the analyst, the object of the transference neurosis.

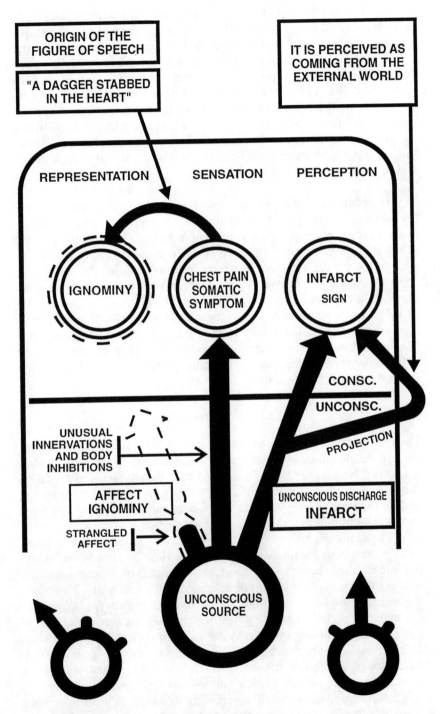

Figure 10

2. In the same way, the actuality of somatic sensations causes them to be transferred in the atemporal present of the session as a false connection with the object "that is there" and is exciting the signs of reality.

3. "Pure" somatic illness, deprived of somatic sensations, is formed according to the principle by which that which is rejected or projected into the world returns as an external perception and is evidenced as an objective alteration (signs) that the patient perceives or ignores. For this reason, somatic illness tends to present itself in the transference–countertransference relationship as an alteration of the setting, a particular and specific distortion of the therapeutic alliance and of the contact with the "real" analyst.

In order that the organ may speak—whether by means of symptoms (sensations) or signs (perceptions)—it is necessary for the psychoanalyst to "counterparticipate in the conversation," by becoming aware of his/her own countertransference, which is tinged with the specificity each of the organs and disorders imposes upon him/her. In the case of somatic sensations, the analyst carries out his/her task holding close to the principles of standard technique, but when he/she is dealing with "pure" somatic sensations, he/she must call upon his/her knowledge of "organ fantasies," analogously to the interpretation of universal symbols in dreams. In his/her everyday practice, the analyst will usually have to be content with restricting interpretation to the territory of secondary resignifications investing those fantasies.

IX. Summary

The German term *Sprache* as well as its English equivalent, "speech," convey the meanings of "code" and *parole* included in the Spanish term *lenguaje* ("language) and its French and Italian equivalents. By the term "code" we allude to a system of signs which may or may not be verbal, and by the term *parole* we refer to the particular act by which we put such a system into practice.

The expression *Organsprache* is used only once by Freud in his 1915 paper about the unconscious (1915e). Here he stated that schizophrenic utterance becomes organ-speech as a result of its acquisition (by means of a somatic sensation) of a "hypochondriacal trait." Therefore, the term *Organsprache* refers unequivocally to a specific type of *Sprache*, or language, performed through the organs and also, that which the organs perform. The organs, like hysterical symptoms (Breuer & Freud, 1895d; Freud, 1896b, 1918b), can "join in the conversation" (*mitsprechen*) by means of symptoms and signs which derive from their alterations. Freud (Breuer & Freud, 1895d) pointed out that hysteria restores the original meaning of the word in depicting its strong innervations when it revives those somatic sensations to which the linguistic expression owes its justification.[4] He finally stated that the hysterical symptom may not have taken the linguistic usage as an archetype, but that both symptom and usage draw their material from a common source. In other papers (1905d, 1915a) Freud asserted that "*any* organ" can function as an erotogenic zone—that is, not only the skin and the mucous membranes, but also the internal organs; by examining the aims of a drive, we can infer its source.[5] The common source mentioned above is, in psychoanalytic theory, an erotogenic zone. Qualitatively differentiated, excitation arises from an erotogenic zone and is capable of reaching consciousness as a definite somatic sensation (dysphagia, for instance) or as a specific cathexis of preconscious word-representations which constitute the linguistic expression or figure of speech, as in the example mentioned above, "to have to swallow an insult."

---

[4]In taking a verbal expression literally and in feeling the "stab in the heart" or "the slap in the face" after some slighting remark as a real event, the hysteric is not taking liberties with words but is simply reviving once more the sensations to which the verbal expression owes its justification. How has it come about that we speak of someone who has been slighted as "being stabbed in the heart" unless the slight had in fact been accompanied by a precordial sensation which could suitably be described in that phrase and unless it was identifiable by that sensation? What could be more probable than that the figure of speech "swallowing something," which we use in talking of an insult to which no rejoinder has been made, in fact originated from the innervatory sensations which arise in the pharynx when we refrain from speaking and prevent ourselves from reacting to the insult? All these sensations and innervations belong to the field of "The expression of the emotions," which, as Darwin has taught us, consists of actions which originally had a meaning and served a purpose. These may now for the most part have become so much weakened that the expression of them in words seems to us only to be a figurative picture of them, whereas in all probability the description was once meant literally; and hysteria is right in restoring the original meaning of the words in depicting its unusually strong innervations. Indeed, it is perhaps wrong to say that hysteria creates those sensations by symbolization. It may be that it does not take linguistic usage as its model at all, but that both hysteria and linguistic usage alike draw their material from a common source (Freud & Breuer, 1895d, p. 181).

[5]It seems probable that any part of the skin and any sense-organ—probably, indeed, *any* organ—can function as an erotogenic zone. . . . It further appears that sexual excitation arises as a by-product, as it were, of a large number of processes that occur in the organism, as soon as they reach a certain degree of intensity . . . (Freud, 1905d, p. 233).

REFERENCES

Abadi, M. (1968), Conferencia en al CIMP, Buenos Aires. Citado por Noemi Canteros en *Contribuciones al Estudio Asma bronquial*. [Conference held at CIMP. Cited by Noemi Canteros in *Contributions to the study of bronchial asthme*.] Buenos Aires: CIMP.

Aberastury, A. (1951), *El Juego de Construir Casas* [The game of building houses]. Buenos Aires: Paidós, 1961.

——— (1971), La dentición, la marcha y el lenguaje. En: *Aportaciones al Psicoanálisis de Niños* [Dentition, walking and language. In: *Contributions to the psychoanalysis of children*]. Buenos Aires: Paidós, pp. 11–29.

——— and Salas, E. (1978), *La Paternidad* [Paternity]. Buenos Aires: Kargieman.

Aeschylus (undated), *The Plays of Aeschylus*. Chicago: University of Chicago Press, 1990.

Aizenberg, S. (1975), La interpretación psicoanalítica. Consideraciones metapsicológicas. [The psychoanalytical interpretation. Metapsychological considerations]. *Eidon* [Buenos Aires], 4:11–29.

Altman, A., and Cattaneo, S. (1978), Algunos rasgos del Carácter varicoso. En: *Jornadas Sobre el Enfermo Cardiovascular* [Some features of the varicose character. In: *Proceedings of a Meeting on the Subject of the Cardiovascular Patient*]. Buenos Aires: CIMP, pp. 96–98.

American Heritage Dictionary of the English Language (1992), ed. 3. Boston: Houghton Mifflin Company, 1996.

Anzieu, D. (1987), *El Yo Piel* [The skin ego]. Madrid: Biblioteca Nueva.

Arana Iñiguez, R., and Rebollo, M. A. (1954), *Neuroanatomía* [Neuroanatomy]. Buenos Aires: El Ateneo, 1960.

Azcoaga, J. (1983), *Las Funciones cerebrales superiores y sus Alteraciones en el Niño y en el Adulto* [Higher brain functions and their alterations in the child and in the adult]. Buenos Aires: Paidós.

Barcia, R. (1961), *Sinónimos castellanos* [Spanish synonyms]. Buenos Aires: Sopena.

Barrow, D. W. (1948), *The Clinical Management of Varicose Veins*. New York: Hoeber, 1957.

Bartleson, D. (1983), Transient and persistent neurological manifestation of migraine. *Stroke*, 15:383–386.

177

Bateson, G. (1979), *Espíritu y Naturaleza* [Mind and nature]. Buenos Aires: Amorrortu.

Bick, E. (1968), La experiencia de la piel en las relaciones de objeto tempranas [Experiences of the skin in early object relations]. *Internat. J. Psychoanalysis*, 49:23 [also *Revista de Psicoanálisis* (Buenos Aires)], 1970, 27:111–117].

Blakeslee, T. R. (1980), *The Right Brain*. New York: Ambos Press.

Blanquez Fraile, A. (1960), *Diccionario Latino-Español* [Latin-Spanish dictionary]. Barcelona: Sopena.

Bleger, J. (1967), *Simbiosis y Ambiguedad* [Symbiosis and ambiguity]. Buenos Aires: Paidós, 1970.

Brenner, C., Friedman, A. P., and Carter, S. (1949), Psychologic factors in the etiology and treatment of chronic headache. *Chronic Headache*, 11:53–56.

Cagnoni, J. (1971), Interpretación psicoanalítica sobra la Función respiratoria. Trabajo presentado en el CIMP. [Psychoanalytic interpretation of the respiratory function. Paper presented at CIMP.] Buenos Aires.

Caino, N., and Sanchez, R. (1978), *Semiología u Orientación diagnóstica de las Enfermedades cardiovasculares* [Semiology or diagnostic orientation in cardiovascular diseases]. Buenos Aires: Panamericana.

Canteros, N. (1979), Contribuciónes al estudio del asma bronquial. Trabajo presentado en el CIMP. [Contributions to the study of bronchial asthma. Paper presented at CIMP.] Buenos Aires.

Cárcamo, C. (1944), *Contribución psicoanalítica al Conocimiento de la Jaqueca. Patología psicosomática* [Psychoanalytical contribution to the knowledge of migraine. Psychosomatic pathology]. Buenos Aires: A.P.A. [Argentine Psychoanalytical Association], 1948.

Cecil, R. & Loeb (1972), *A Textbook of Medicine*. Philadelphia: Saunders.

Cesio, F. (1960), El Letargo. Contribución al estudio de la RTN. En: *Un Estudio del Hombre que Padece* [Lethargy. Contribution to the study of negative therapeutic reaction. In: *A Study of the Man that Suffers*]. Buenos Aires: Kargieman, pp. 41–52.

Chiozza, L. (1963), *Psicoanálisis de los Trastornos Hepáticos* [Psychoanalysis of hepatic disorders, preliminary communication]. Buenos Aires: Luro.

——— (1970), *Psicoanálisis de los Trastornos Hepáticos* [Psychoanalysis of hepatic disorders]. Buenos Aires: Kargieman.

——— (1970a), Apuntes sobre fantasía, materia y lenguaje. En: *Trama y Figura del Enfermar y del Psicoanalizar* [Notes on fantasy, matter and language. In: *Weft and Figure in Falling Ill and Psychoanalyzing*]. Buenos Aires: Paidós, 1980, pp. 117–125.

——— (1971), Las fantasías específicas en la investigación psicoanalítica de la relación psique y soma. En: *Trama y figura del Enfermar y del Psicoanalizar* [Specific fantasies in psychoanalytic investigation in the psyche-soma relation. In: *Weft and Figure in Falling Ill and Psychoanalyzing*]. Buenos Aires: Paidós, 1980, pp. 125–137.

—— (1971a), La interioridad de lo inconsciente. En: *Periódico Informativo* [The interiorness of the unconscious. In: *Information Journal* (Buenos Aires: CIMP)]. 4:17–19.

—— (1972), Conocimiento y acto en medicina psicosomática. En: *Trama y Figura del Enfermar y del Psicoanalizar* [Knowledge and act in psychosomatic medicine. In: *Weft and Figure in Falling Ill and Psychoanalyzing*]. Buenos Aires: Paidós, 1980, pp. 197–217.

—— (1974), La transformación del afecto en lenguaje. En: *Trama y Figura del Enfermar y del Psicoanalizar* [The transformation of affect into language. In: *Weft and Figure in Falling Ill and Psychoanalyzing*]. Buenos Aires: Paidós, 1980, pp. 217–227.

—— (1974b), Estudio psicoanalítico de las fantasías hepáticas. En: *Trama y Figura del Enfermar y del Psicoanalizar* [Psychoanalytical study of hepatic fantasies. In: *Weft and Figure in Falling Ill and Psychoanalyzing*]. Buenos Aires: Paidós, 1980, pp. 87–116.

—— (1976), Cuerpo, Afecto y Lenguaje [*Body, Affect and Language*]. Buenos Aires: Paidós.

—— (1976a), La enfermedad de los afectos. En: *Trama y Figura del Enfermar y del Psicoanalizar* [The Illness of affects. In: *Weft and Figure in Falling Ill and Psychoanalyzing*]. Buenos Aires: Paidós, 1980, pp. 245–257.

—— (1978), El corazón tiene razones que la razón ignora. En: *Trama y Figura del Enfermar y del Psicoanalizar* [The heart has reasons that reason ignores. In: *Weft and Figure in Falling Ill and Psychoanalyzing*]. Buenos Aires: Paidós, 1980, pp. 357–363.

—— (1978a), El problema de la simbolización en la enfermedad somática. En: *Trama y Figura del Enfermar y del Psicoanalizar* [The problem of symbolization in somatic illness. In: *Weft and Figure in Falling Ill and Psychoanalyzing*]. Buenos Aires: Paidós, 1980, pp. 293–349.

—— (1980), *Trama y Figura del Enfermar y del Psicoanalizar* [*Weft and Figure in Falling Ill and Psychoanalyzing*]. Buenos Aires: Paidós.

—— (1980a), Corazón, hígado y cerebro. Introducción esquemática a la comprensión de un trilema. En: *Psicoanálisis: Presente y Futuro* [Heart, liver and brain. Schematic introduction to the comprehension of a conflict triggered by a triple motto. In: *Psychoanalysis: Present and Future*]. Buenos Aires: CIMP, 1983, pp. 103–115.

—— (1981), Entre la nostalgia y el anhelo. Un ensayo acerca de la vinculación entre la noción de tiempo y la melancolía. En: *Psicoanálisis: Presente y Futuro* [Between nostalgia and yearning. Essay about the relation between the notion of time and melancholia. In: *Psychoanalysis: Present and Future*]. Buenos Aires: Paidós, 1983, pp. 115–127.

—— (1981a), La capacidad simbólica de la estructura y el funcionamiento del cuerpo [Symbolic capacity of the structure and functioning of the body]. *Eidon* [Buenos Aires], 15:45–61.

—— (1984), *Psicoanálisis de los Trastornos Hepáticos* [Psychoanalysis of hepatic disorders]. Buenos Aires: CIMP.

——— (1986), *¿Por Qué Enfermamos?* [Why do we fall ill?] Buenos Aires: Alianza (English edition, in press).

——— (1986a), Un infarto en lugar de una ignominia. En: *¿Por Qué Enfermamos?* [An infarct instead of ignominy. In: *Why Do We Fall Ill?*] Buenos Aires: Alianza, pp. 76–88 (English edition, in press).

——— (1986b), Estudio psicoanalítico de las ampollas. En: *¿Por Qué Enfermamos?* [Psychoanalytical study of blisters. In: *Why Do We Fall Ill?*] Buenos Aires: Alianza, pp. 97–98 (English edition, in press).

——— (1986c), La sangre tira. En: *¿Por Qué Enfermamos?* [Blood is thicker than water. In: *Why Do We Fall Ill?*] Buenos Aires: Alianza, pp. 127–138 (English edition, in press).

——— (1986d), Un lunar inocente. En: *¿Por Qué Enfermamos?* [An innocent mole. In: *Why Do We Fall Ill?*] Buenos Aires: Alianza, pp. 99–112 (English edition, in press).

——— (1989), *Organsprache*, quaderni di psicoterapia infantile. Rome: Borla, 1991, 23:15–44, and in Luis Chiozza and André Green, *Diálogo Psicoanalítico Sobre Psicosomática* [Psychoanalytic Dialogue on Psychosomatics]. Buenos Aires: Alianza, 1952, pp. 19–46.

——— Aizenberg, S., Califano, C., Fonzi, A., Grus, R., Obstfeld, J., Sainz, J., and Scapusio, J. C. (1982), Las cardiopatías isquémicas. Patobiografía de un enfermo de ignominia. En: *Psicoanálisis: Presente y Futuro* [Ischemic cardiopathy. Pathobiography of a person suffering from ignominy. In: *Psychoanalysis: Present and Future*]. Buenos Aires: Paidós, 1983, pp. 287–323.

——— Califano, C., Korovsky, E., Malfé, R., Turjansky, D., and Wainer, G. (1964), Una idea de la lágrima. En: *Trama y Figura del Enfermar y del Psicoanalizar* [An idea of the tear. In: *Weft and Figure in Falling Ill and Psychoanalyzing*]. Buenos Aires: Paidós, 1980, pp. 137–167.

——— Laborde, V., Obstfeld, E., and Pantolini, J. (1966), Estudio y desarrollo de algunos conceptos de Freud acerca del interpretar. En: *Un Estudio del Hombre que Padece* [Study and development of some Freudian concepts about interpreting. In: *A Study of the Man That Suffers*]. Buenos Aires: CIMP-Kargieman, 1978, pp. 271–291.

——— Baldino, O., Carotenuto, L., Funosas, M., and Obstfeld, E. (1987), Las fantasias específicas de los trastornos respiratorios. Communicación preliminar. Trabajo presentado en el CIMP. [The specific fantasies of the respiratory disorders. Paper presented at CIMP.] Buenos Aires.

Civita, V., Ed. (1973), *Atlas de Biología* [Biology atlas]. Barcelona: Salvat, 1974.

Cobb, S. (1954), *Fundamentos de Neuropsiquiatría* [The Basis of Neuropsychiatry]. Buenos Aires: Swescun-Barrenechea.

Collins, W. (1987), *English Language Dictionary*. London: Harper-Collins, 1993.

Corominas, J. (1961), *Breve Diccionario etimológico de la Lengua Castellana* [Concise etymological dictionary of the Spanish language]. Madrid: Gredos, 1983.

Cremerius, J. (1956), El significado de la oralidad en la diabetes senil y en la fase depresiva relacionada con la misma, discurso aniversario de la Sociedad Alemana de Psicoterapia y Psicologia Profunda [The meaning of orality in senile diabetes and the depressive stage related to it. Anniversary Speech at the German Society of Psychotherapy and Depth Psychology]. *Psicosomática Clínica*. Borla: Rome, 1981, pp. 193–208.

Daniels, G. E. (1936), Analysis of a case of neurosis with diabetes mellitus. *Psychoanal. Quart.*, 5:513–547.

Daniels, L. (1964), *Pruebas Funcionales musculares* [Muscular functional tests]. Buenos Aires: Interamericana.

Darwin, C. (1872), *The Expression of Emotions in Man and Animals*. London: Dover, N. H. and F. Pinter, 1983.

Del Campo Llerena, A. (1984), *Patología venosa* [Venous pathology]. Buenos Aires: Intermédica.

Del Sel, J. M. (1963), *Ortopedia y Traumatología* [Orthopedics and traumatology]. Buenos Aires: López, 1979.

De Miguel, R., and Marqués de Morante (1943), *Diccionario Etimológico Latino-Español*, ed. 23 [Latin-Spanish Etymological Dictionary]. Madrid: Librería General Victoriano Suárez.

de Saussure, F. (1945), *Curso de Linguística general* [Course in general linguistics]. Buenos Aires: Losada.

Diccionario Enciclopédico Hispano-Americano (1912), [Spanish-American dictionary]. Madrid: Montaner & Simon.

Diccionario Etimológico de la Lengua alemana (1963), [Etymological dictionary of the German language]. Mannheim: Dudenverlag.

Diccionario Sapiens (1954), [Sapiens dictionary]. Buenos Aires: Sopena.

Dorland's Diccionario de Ciencias Médicas [Dorland's dictionary of medical sciences]. Barcelona: El Ateneo, 1983.

Dostoievsky, F. (1864), *Memorias del Subsuelo* [Notes from underground]. Buenos Aires: Jorge Alvarez, 1969.

Dumas, G. (1933), *Nuevo Tratado de Psicología*, vol. III [New psychology treatise]. Buenos Aires: Kapelusz, 1950.

Dunbar, H. F., Wolfe, T., and Rioch, J. M. (1936), Psychiatric aspect of medical disorders. Psychic component of the process of disease in cardiac, diabetic and fracture patients. *Amer. J. Psychiat.*, 93:649–679.

Eckersley, C. E. (1960), *A Comprehensive English Grammar*. London: Longmans.

Eliade, M. (1955), *Imágenes y Símbolos* [Images and symbols]. Madrid: Taurus, 1974.

——— (1964), *Tratado de Historia de las Religiones* [Treatise on the history of religions]. Madrid: Cristiandad, 1974.

Enciclopedia Salvat (1972), Barcelona: Salvat.

——— (1985), *Diccionario de Ciencias Médicas*, ed. 12. [Dictionary of medical sciences]. Barcelona: Salvat.

——— (1986), *Diccionario enciclopédico* [Encyclopedic dictionary]. Barcelona: Salvat.

Ernout, A., and Meillet, A. (1959), *Dictionaire etymologique de la Langue latine* [Etymological dictionary of the Latin language]. París: Klicksiek.

Etcheverry, J. L. (1978), *Sobre la Versión castellana* [On the Spanish version]. Buenos Aires: Amorrortu, 1978.

Ey, H., Bernard, P., Brisset, Ch. (1965), *Tratado de Psiquiatría* [Treatise of psychiatry]. Barcelona: Toray Masson, 1969.

Farber, E., and Van Scott, E. (1980), Psoriasis. En: *Dermatología en Medicina General* [Psoriasis. In: *Dermatology in General Medicine*]. Buenos Aires: Médica Panamericana.

Farreras Valenti, P., and Rozman, C. (1982), *Medicina Interna* [Internal medicine]. Barcelona: Marín, 1984.

Fenichel, O. (1957), *Teoría general de las Neurosis* [The psychoanalytic theory of neurosis. New York: W. W. Norton]. Buenos Aires: Nova, 1957.

Ferguson, M. (1983), *La Revolución du Cervau* [The revolution of the brain]. Ed. Calmann-Levy. Paris: 1974.

Ferrater Mora, J. (1954), *Diccionario de Filosofía* [Dictionary of philosophy]. Buenos Aires: Sudamericana, 1958.

Fitzpatrick, T., Eisen, A., Wolff, K., Freedberg, Y., and Austen, K. F. (1979), *Dermatología en Medicina General* [Dermatology in general medicine]. Buenos Aires: Médica Panamericana, 1980.

Foks, G., Alperovich, J., Navedo, R., Rodriguez, F., and Satke, R. (1969), La piel. Observaciones sobre una fantasía específica [Skin. Observations concerning a specific fantasy]. *I Symposium*. Buenos Aires: CIMP, pp. 164–169.

Foote, R. R. (1969), *Venas Varicosas. Manual Práctico* [Varicose veins. Practical handbook]. Buenos Aires: Ed. López Libreros.

Fracassi, H. (1945), *Vías de Conducción de la Energéa nerviosa* [Ways of conduction of nervous energy]. Córdoba, Argentina: Imprenta de la Universidad.

French, T., and Alexander, F. (1960), *Psicología y asma bronquial* [Psychogenic factors in bronchial asthma]. Buenos Aires: Paidós, 1960.

Freud, S. (1895b), On the grounds for detaching a particular syndrome from neurasthenia under the description "anxiety neurosis." *Standard Edition*, 3:87–117. London: Hogarth Press, 1962.

——— (1896b), Further remarks on the neuro-psychoses of defence. *Standard Edition*, 3:159–185. London: Hogarth Press, 1962.

——— (1900a), The interpretation of dreams. *Standard Edition*, 4:1–338, 5:339–751. London: Hogarth Press, 1953.

——— (1901b), The psychopathology of everyday life. *Standard Edition*, 6:1–279. London: Hogarth Press, 1960.

——— (1905d), Three essays on the theory of sexuality. *Standard Edition*, 7:123–245. London: Hogarth Press, 1953.

——— (1905e), Fragment of an analysis of a case of hysteria. *Standard Edition*, 7:1–122. London: Hogarth Press, 1953.

———— (1909a), Some general remarks on hysterical attacks. *Standard Edition*, 9:227–234. London: Hogarth Press, 1959.

———— (1910a), Five lectures on psycho-analysis. *Standard Edition*, 11:1–56. London: Hogarth Press, 1957.

———— (1910e), The antithetical meaning of primal words. *Standard Edition*, 11:153–161. London: Hogarth Press, 1957.

———— (1910i), The psycho-analytic view of psychogenic disturbance of vision. *Standard Edition*, 11:209–218. London: Hogarth Press, 1957.

———— (1911b), Formulations on the two principles of mental functioning. *Standard Edition*, 12:215. London: Hogarth Press, 1958.

———— (1911c), Psycho-analytic notes on an autobiographical account of a case of paranoia [Dementia paranoides]. *Standard Edition*, 12:11–82. London: Hogarth Press, 1958.

———— (1912e), Recommendations to physicians practising psycho-analysis. *Standard Edition*, 12:109–120. London: Hogarth Press, 1958.

———— (1912f), Contributions to a discussion on masturbation. *Standard Edition*, 12:239–254. London: Hogarth Press, 1958.

———— (1912–1913), Totem and taboo. *Standard Edition*, 13:1–162. London: Hogarth Press, 1955.

———— (1913i), The disposition to obsessional neurosis: A contribution to the problem of choice of neurosis. *Standard Edition*, 12:317–326. London: Hogarth Press, 1958.

———— (1913j), The claims of psycho-analysis to scientific interest. *Standard Edition*, 13:163–190. London: Hogarth Press, 1955.

———— (1914c), On narcissism: An introduction. *Standard Edition*, 14:67–102. London: Hogarth Press, 1957.

———— (1915a), Observations on transference-love (Further recommendations on the technique of psycho-analysis, III). *Standard Edition*, 12:159–171. London: Hogarth Press, 1958.

———— (1915b), Thoughts for the times on war and death. *Standard Edition*, 14:275–300. London: Hogarth Press, 1958.

———— (1915c), Instincts and their vicissitudes. *Standard Edition*, 14:109–140. London: Hogarth Press, 1957.

———— (1915e), The unconscious. *Standard Edition*, 14:159–215. London: Hogarth Press, 1957.

———— (1916–1917), Introductory lectures on psycho-analysis. *Standard Edition*, 15:1–239. London: Hogarth Press, 1961; 16:241–463. London: Hogarth Press, 1963.

———— (1917d), A metapsychological supplement to the theory of dreams. *Standard Edition*, 14:217–235. London: Hogarth Press, 1957.

———— (1918b), From the history of an infantile neurosis. *Standard Edition*, 17:1–122. London: Hogarth Press, 1955.

———— (1920g), Beyond the pleasure principle. *Standard Edition*, 18:1–64. London: Hogarth Press, 1955.

———— (1923a), Two encyclopaedia articles. *Standard Edition*, 18:233–259. London: Hogarth Press, 1955.

———— (1923b), The ego and the id. *Standard Edition*, 19:1–62. London: Hogarth Press, 1961.

———— (1924c), The economic problem of masochism. *Standard Edition*, 19:155–170. London: Hogarth Press, 1961.

———— (1926d), Inhibitions, symptoms and anxiety. *Standard Edition*, 20:75–175. London: Hogarth Press, 1959.

———— (1930a), Civilization and its discontents. *Standard Edition*, 21:57–145. London: Hogarth Press, 1961.

———— (1933a), New introductory lectures on psycho-analysis, *Standard Edition*, 22:1–182. London: Hogarth Press, 1964.

———— (1939a), Moses and monotheism. *Standard Edition*, 23:1–137. London: Hogarth Press, 1964.

———— (1940a), An outline of psycho-analysis. *Standard Edition*, 23:139–207. London: Hogarth Press, 1964.

———— (1940b), Some elementary lessons in psycho-analysis. *Standard Edition*, 23:279–286. London: Hogarth Press, 1964.

———— (1940e), Splitting of the ego in the process of defence. *Standard Edition*, 23:271–278. London: Hogarth Press, 1964.

———— (1950a), Extracts from the Fliess papers: [Letter 59. *Standard Edition*, 1:244–245. Letter 102. *Standard Edition*, 1:277–278. Project for a scientific psychology. *Standard Edition*, 1:283–397. Draft I.: Migraine: Established points. *Standard Edition*, 1:213–215.] London: Hogarth Press, 1966.

———— with Breuer, J. (1895d), Studies on hysteria. *Standard Edition*, 2:1–309. London: Hogarth Press, 1955.

———— and Bullit, W. (1966), Introduction to S. Freud and W. C. Bullit, *Thomas Woodrow Wilson, Twenty-Eighth President of the United States: A Psychological Study*. London: Weidenfeld and Nicholson, 1967.

Garma, A. (1940), *Psicoanálisis de los Sueños* [Psychoanalysis of dreams]. Buenos Aires: Ateneo.

———— (1954), *Génesis psicosomática y Tratamiento de las úlceras gástricas y duodenales* [Psychosomatic genesis and treatment of gastric and duodenal ulcer]. Buenos Aires: Nova.

———— (1956), "Los sueños son alucinaciones de situaciones traumáticas enmascaradas" [Dreams are hallucinations of disguised traumatic situations]. *Revista de Psicoanálisis*, 4, Buenos Aires, pp. 397–402.

———— (1958), *El Dolor de Cabeza* [Headache]. Buenos Aires: Nova.

———— (1961), *Psicoanálisis del Arte ornamental* [Psychoanalysis of ornamental art]. Buenos Aires: Paidós.

———— (1969), *El Psicoanálisis–Teoría, Clínica y Técnica* [Psychoanalysis–theory, clinic and technique]. Buenos Aires: Paidós, 1971.

———— (1970), *Nuevas Aportaciones al Psicoanálisis de los Sueños* [New contributions to psychoanalysis on dreams]. Buenos Aires: Paidós.

—— (1972), *Psicoanálisis del Dolor de Cabeza* [Psychoanalysis of the headache]. Buenos Aires: Paidós.

—— (1975), Comentario al trabajo de E. Obstfeld, "El diabetico: un hombre insatisfecho," presentado en el CIMP. [Commentary on the paper "The diabetic: an unsatisfied man," presented by E. Obstfeld at CIMP.] Buenos Aires.

Gatti, J. C., and Cardama, J. E. (1963), *Manual de Dermatología* [Dermatology handbook]. Buenos Aires: El Ateneo.

Gelmers, H. (1985), Calcium-channel blockers in the treatment of migraine. *Amer. J. Cardiol.*, 55:139–143.

Granel, J. (1975), Hacia una teoría de los accidentes [Towards a theory of accidents]. *Eidón* [Buenos Aires: CIMP, Paidós], 4:29–44.

Graves, R. (1960), *The Greek Myths*, vols. 1 and 2. New York: Penguin Books.

Greenburg, D. (1969), *Cómo Ser una idische Mame* [How to be a Jewish mother]. Buenos Aires: Hormé.

Griffero, E. (1982), *Príncipe Azul, Cuadernos* [Prince Charming]. Buenos Aires: Wd. Adans, 1984.

Grimal, P. (1963), *Mitologías de las Estepas, de los Bosques y de las Islas* [Mythologies of the steppes, the woods and the islands]. Barcelona: Planeta, 1973.

—— (1981), *Diccionario de Mitología griega y romana* [Dictionary of Greek and Roman mythology]. Buenos Aires: Paidós.

Grimm, the Brothers (1974), Hansel y Gretel. En: *Cuentos de Hadas* [Hansel and Gretel. In: *Fairy Tales*]. Buenos Aires: ACME.

Gur, R. R., and Gur, R. C. (1975), Defense mechanisms. Psychosomatic symptomatology and conjugate lateral eye movements. *Consult. and Clinical Psych.*, 43:416–420.

Guyton, A. C. (1971), *Textbook of Medical Physiology*, ed. 4. Philadelphia: Saunders.

Ham-Leeson (1963), *Tratado de Histología* [Histology treatise]. Mexico City: Interamericana.

Harrison, T. R. (1962), *Principles of Internal Medicine*. New York: McGraw-Hill.

Houssay, B. (1955), *Fisiología humana* [Human physiology]. Buenos Aires: Ateneo, 1958.

Hoyle, F., and Wickramasinghe, N. C. (1978), *Lifecloud. The Origin of Life in the Universe*. London: Dent, 1981.

Jerne, N. K. (1973), The immune system. In: *The Harvey Lectures*. London: Academic Press, 1975.

Jimenez Diaz, C. (1936), *Lecciones de Patología médica* [Lectures on medical pathology]. Barcelona: Científica Médica.

Jones, E. (1953–1957), *Vida y Obra de Sigmund Freud* [Life and work of Sigmund Freud. New York: Basic Books]. Buenos Aires: Hormé, 1979.

Kimura, D. (1973), *L'Asimmetria del Cervello umano* [The asymmetry of the human brain]. Milano: Scienze, 1978.

Klein, M. (1954), Notes on some schizoid mechanisms. In: *Developments in Psychoanalysis*. London: Hogarth Press, pp. 292–320.

———— Heimann, P., Isaacs, S., and Riviere, J. (1952), Some theoretical conclusions regarding the emotional life of the infant. In: *Developments in Psychoanalysis*. London: Hogarth Press, pp. 198–236.

Korovsky, E. (1978), Aportes para la comprensión de la psoriasis [Contributions to the understanding of psoriasis]. *IX Symposium*. Buenos Aires: CIMP, pp. 135–139.

Laborde, V., Aducci, E., Canteros, N. L. de, Devicenzi, A., Mariona, A., and Wainer, G. (1973), *La Sangre. Una Approximación al Comocimiento sobre su Fantasia específica* [The blood. An approximation to knowledge of its specific fantasy]. Buenos Aires: CIMP.

Lacour, R. (1981), *Insuficiencia venosa en los Miembros inferiores* [Venous insufficiency of the lower limbs]. Buenos Aires: El Ateneo.

Laplanche, J., and Pontalis, B. (1967), *Vocabulaire de la Psychanalyse* [Vocabulary of psychoanalysis]. París: Presses Universitaires de France.

Leao, A. A. P. (1944), Spreading depression of activity in cerebral cortex. In: Campbell, J. K., and Caselli, R. J., Eds., *Headache and Cranio-facial pain in Neurology in Clinical Practice*. Bradley, Walter G. Newton, MA, 1996, pp. 1683–1719.

Lechin, F., and Van der Dijs, B. (1980), Physiological, clinical and therapeutical basis of a new hypothesis for headache. *Headache J.*, 202:27–84.

Lorenz, K. (1976), Las bases innatas del aprendizaje. En: *Biología del Aprendizaje*, compilado por Pribram [The innate bases of apprenticeship. In: *Biology of Apprenticeship*, compiled by Pribram]. Buenos Aires: Paidós.

Lovelock, J. E. (1979), *Gaia. Una nueva Visión sobre la Tierra* [Gaia. A new look at life on earth]. Madrid: Blume, 1983.

Mac Lean, P. D. (1984), *Evoluzione del Cervello e Comportamento umano* [Evolution of the brain and human behavior]. Torino: Ed. G. Einaudi.

Magnin, P. H. (1977), *Dermatología en el Pregrado* [Undergraduate dermatology]. Buenos Aires: López.

Menninger, K. (1935), Interrelationships of mental disorders and diabetes mellitus. *J. Mental. Sc.*, 81:332–357.

Merriam-Webster's Dictionary of English Usage (1989), ed. 10. Springfield, MA: Merriam-Webster.

Miller De Paiva, L. (1966), *Medicina Psicosomática* [Psychosomatic medicine]. San Pablo: Librería Editora Arts Medical.

Moliner, M. (1986), *Diccionario del Uso español* [Dictionary of Spanish usage]. Madrid: Gredos.

Morales Macedo, C. (1955), *Biología fundamental* [Fundamental biology]. Barcelona: Salvat.

Morris, D. (1977), *El Hombre al Desnudo* [Man in his naked condition]. Barcelona: Nauta, 1980.

Murray, J. F. (1983), Crecimiento y desarrollo del aparato respiratorio. En: Smith, L., and Tier, S. O., Eds., *Fisiopatología, Principios biológicos de la Enfermedad* [Growth and development of the respiratory system. In: *Physiopathology, Biologic Principles of Disease*]. Buenos Aires: Médica Panamericana.

Noyes, A. (1951), *Modern Clinical Psychiatry*. Philadelphia: Saunders.

Oakley, G., Pike, D. A., and Taylor, K. W. (1974), *Diabetes y su Tratamiento* [Diabetes and its treatment]. Buenos Aires: Editorial Bernardes.

Obermayer, M. (1956), *Medicina Psicocutánea* [Psychocutaneous medicine]. Buenos Aires: Bibliográfica Argentina.

Obstfeld, E. (1970), Notas para un carácter diabético. [Notes on a diabetic character]. *II Symposium*. Buenos Aires: CIMP, pp. 1–7.

———— (1971), El mito de Tántalo. Su comprensión a la luz de las fantasías diabéticas [The myth of Tantalus. Its meaning in the light of diabetic fantasies]. *Periódico informativo del CIMP* [Buenos Aires], 2:29–32.

———— (1975), Psicoanálisis del trastorno diabético [Psychoanalysis of the diabetic disorder]. *Eidon* [Buenos Aires: Paidós], 5:33–59, 6:83–88, 1976.

———— (1978), Jornadas sobre el enfermo cardiovascular [Some ideas about the cardiovascular patient] presented at the Seminar on the Cardiovascular Patient. Symposium (publication). Buenos Aires: CIMP, pp. 37–41.

———— (1988), Significado y uso de los afectos del analista frente al paciente "somático," Revista A.P.A. [Meaning and use of the analyst's affects in relation to the "somatic" patient]. *Journal of Argentine Psychoanalytical Association* [Buenos Aires], 45:1037–1046.

————, Bahamonde, C., de Eliano, L., de Erbin, S., Litvinoff, N., de Litvinoff, E., de Rotblat, N., and Scapusio, J. C. (1975), Comprensión psicoanalítica del trastorno pulmonar [The psychoanalytic comprehension of the pulmonary disorder]. *Eidon* [Buenos Aires: Paidós.], 2:83–92.

————, Baldino, O., Dayen, E., Marín, E., Rodriguez, C., Salzman, R., and Santalla, J. (1983a), Lo respiratorio en la literatura [The respiratory subject in literature]. *XIV Simposio del CIMP*. Buenos Aires: CIMP, pp. 119–123.

————, ————, ————, ————, ————, ————, and ———— (1983b), Lo respiratorio y la creación [The respiratory subject and creation]. *IX Simposio del CIMP*. Buenos Aires: CIMP, pp. 124–130.

————, ————, and Salzman, R. (1982), El desgano y la relación psicoanalítica [Dispiritedness and the psychoanalytic relation]. *XIII Simposio del CIMP*. Buenos Aires: CIMP, pp. 76–81.

Odisio, A. (1979), *Várices de los Miembros inferiores* [The varicose veins of the lower limbs]. Buenos Aires: Akadia.

Olesen, J., Larsen, B., and Lauritzen, M. (1981), Focal hyperemia followed by spreading oligemia and impaired activation of VCBF in classic migraine. *Ann. Neurol.*, 9:344–352.

Osterrieth, P. (1973), *Psicología infantil* [Infant psychology]. Madrid: Morata.

Panconesi, E., Ammon, G., Cossidente, A., Finke, G., Giorgini, S., Herold, Y., Marzi, C., Melli, C., Messeri, P., Montagu, A., Pasini, W., Petrini, N., Sarti, M., Shanon, J., Schibalski-Ammon, K., and Tassinari, G. (1984), *Stress and Skin Diseases: Psychosomatic Dermatology*. Philadelphia: Lippincott.

Papaleo, O. (1975), Comentario al trabajo "El diabético: un hombre insatisfecho," presentado en el primer Encuentro Argentino-Brasileño. Contribuciónes a la Medicina Psicosomática. [Commentary on the paper "The diabetic: an unsatisfied man," presented at the first Argentine-Brazilian Encounter. Contributions to Psychosomatic Medicine.] Buenos Aires.

Partridge, E. (1966), *Origins*. London: Routledge and Kegan Paul.

——— (1966a), *A Short Etymological Dictionary of Modern English*. New York: Macmillan.

Paz, O. (1956), *El Arco y la Lira* [The bow and the lyre]. México: Fondo de Cultura Económica, 1983.

Perez Rioja, J. A. (1962), *Diccionario de Símbolos y Mitos* [Dictionary of symbols and myths]. Madrid: Tecnos, 1980.

Perrault, C. (1971), *Contes* [Adaptation deux Cogs D'Or]. Paris.

Pichon-Rivière, E. (1943), Los dinamismos de la epilepsia. En: *Del Psicoanálisis a la Psicología Social* [The Dynamisms of epilepsy. In: *From Psychoanalysis to Social Psychology*, E. Pichon-Riviere, ed.]. Buenos Aires: Editorial Ederma, 1970, pp. 115–166.

Pietravallo, A. (1985), *Flebopatías superficiales y profundas* [Superficial and profound phlebopathies]. Buenos Aires: Ciba-Geigy.

Pirandello, L. (1921), *Sei personaggi in cerca d'autore* [Six characters in search of an author]. Milan: Mondadori.

Portmann, A. (1954), Los cambios en el pensamiento biológico. En: *La Nueva Visión del Mundo* [Changes in biological thought. In: *The New View of the World*, ed. Sankt Gallen Institute of Higher Studies]. Buenos Aires: Editorial Sudamericana, 1955.

——— (1961), *Nuevos Caminos de la Biología* [New ways in biology]. Madrid: Iberoamericana, 1968.

Racker, E. (1948), Un caso de impotencia, asma y conducta masoquista [A case of impotence, asthma and masochistic behavior]. *Revista Argentina de Psicoanálisis* [Buenos Aires], 3:578–627.

——— (1958), *Estudios sobre Técnica psicoanalítica* [Studies of psychoanalytic technique]. Buenos Aires: Paidós, 1964.

Random House Dictionary of the English Language (1966), New York, N.Y.

Rascol, A., Cambier, J., Guiraud, B., Manelfe, C., David, J., and Clanet, M. (1979), Accidents ischemiques cerebreaux au cours de crises migraneuses [Ischemic brain accidents during crisis of migraine]. *Revista de Neurología* [Paris], 12:867–884.

Raskin, N. H. (1988), On the origin of head pain. *Headache J.*, 28:254–257.

——— (1988a), On the origin of head pain. The hypnic headache syndrome. *Headache J.*, 28:534–536.

——— (1989), The pathogenesis of migraine (Current opinion in neurology & neurosurgery). *Current Science*, 2.

——— Hosobuchi, Y., and Lamb, S. (1987), Headache may arise from perturbation of brain. *Headache J.*, 27:416–420.

Raskovsky, A. (1960), *El Psiquismo Fetal* [The fetal psyche]. Buenos Aires: Paidós.

Real Academia Española (1950), *Diccionario de la Lengua española* [Dictionary of the Spanish language]. Madrid: Espasa-Calpe, 1985.

Reich, W. (1933), *Análisis del Carácter* [Character analysis]. México: Paidós Mejicana, 1987.

Rof Carballo, J. (1950), *Patología Psicosomática* [Psychosomatic pathology]. Madrid: Paz Montalvo.

Rosenfeld, D. (1975), Trastornos en la piel y el esquema corporal [Disorders of the skin and body scheme]. *Revista de Psicoanálisis*, 32: 309–348.

Ruiz Torres, F. (1959), *Diccionario de Medicina Alemán-Español* [Dictionary of medicine]. Madrid: Alhambra.

Ryan, R., and Ryan, R. (1980), *Cefaleas. Diagnóstico y tratamiento* [Headaches. Diagnosis and treatment]. Buenos Aires: Bernardes.

Sagrada Biblia (undated), Edición Comentada por Nacar, E., y Colunga, A., VIII edición [Sagrada Bible with commentaries by E. Nacar and A. Colunga, ed. 27]. Madrid: Católica, 1968.

Schilder, P. (1958), *Imagen y Apariencia del Cuerpo humano* [Image and appearance of the body]. Buenos Aires: Paidós.

Serrantes, N., and Cardonet, L. (1969), *Diabetes*. Buenos Aires: Médica Panamericana.

Shephard, J., and Vanhoutte, P. (1978), Papel del sistema venoso en el control circulatorio [The function of the venous system in circulatory control]. *Revista de Angiología* [Buenos Aires], 32:247–250.

Skeat, W. (1882), *Concise Dictionary of English Etymology*. Hertfordshire, England: Wordsworth Edition Ltd., 1994.

Solomon, S., Cappa, G., and Smith, Ch. (1988), Common migraine: Criteria for diagnosis. *Headache*, 28:124–129.

Sperry, R. W. (1962), Interhemispheric relations and cerebral dominance. Conference J. Young. Ed. Baltimore: Johns Hopkins University Press.

Stein, J. (1987), *Medicina interna* [Internal medicine]. Buenos Aires: Salvat.

Strandberg, J. (1932), Psique y enfermedades de la piel. En: *Psicogénesis y Psicoterapia de los Síntomas corporales*, by O. Schwarz [Psyche and skin diseases. In: *Psychotherapy and Psychogenesis of Corporal Symptoms*]. Barcelona: Labor, pp. 272–286.

REFERENCES

Swarthy, S. (1939), *Tratado de Mitología* [Treatise on mythology]. Buenos Aires: Araujo, 1939.

Taylor, G. R. (1979), *The Natural History of the Mind*. London: Martin Secker & Warburg, 1981.

Thomas, L. (1974), *Las Vidas de las Células* [The lives of a cell]. Buenos Aires: Emecé, 1976.

Viglioglia, P., and Rubin, J. (1974), *Cosmiatría. Fundamentos científicos y técnicos* [Cosmetology. Scientific and technical basis]. Buenos Aires: E. C., 1979.

Villée, C. (1957), *Biology*. Philadelphia: Saunders.

Vincent, J. D. (1986), *Biologie des Passions* [Biology of the passions]. París: Odile Jacob.

Vogel, G., and Angerman, H. (1974), *Atlas de Biología* [Atlas of biology]. Barcelona: Omega.

Watzlawick, P. (1977), *El Lenguaje del Cambio* [The language of change]. Barcelona: Herder S.A., 1980.

Webster's Collegiate Dictionary (1898), ed. 10. Massachusetts: Merriam Webster, 1996.

Weiss, E., and English, O. (1949), *Medicina Psicosomática* [Psychosomatic medicine]. Buenos Aires: López y Etchegoyen.

Weisz, P. B. (1971), *The Science of Zoology*. New York: McGraw-Hill.

Weizsaecker, V. Von (1950a), *Casos y Problemas clínicos* [Clinical cases and problems]. Barcelona: Pubul.

——— (1950b), *Patosofía* [Pathosophy]. Goettingen: Vandenhoeck & Ruprecht, 1956.

——— (1950c), *El Círculo de la Forma* [The circle of the form]. Madrid: Morata, 1962.

——— (1956), *El Hombre enfermo* [The sick person]. Barcelona: Luis Miracle.

Wisdom, J. O. (1961), Comparación y Desarrollo de las Teorías psicoanalíticas sobre la Melancolía. Fasciculo de Circulación interno de A. P. A., Asociación Psicoanalítica Argentina. [Comparison and development of psychoanalytic theories about melancholia.] Buenos Aires: Asociación Psicoanalítica Argentina, 1966.

Wolff, H. G. (1972), *Headache and Other Head Pain*. New York: Oxford University Press.

Wyss, W. (1947), *Cuerpo y Espíritu* [Body and spirit]. Barcelona: Manuel Marin, 1974.

Ziegler, A. (1986), *Emicrania e Bestialitá* [Migraine and bestiality]. *Riza Psicosomática* [Milan], 67:52–57.